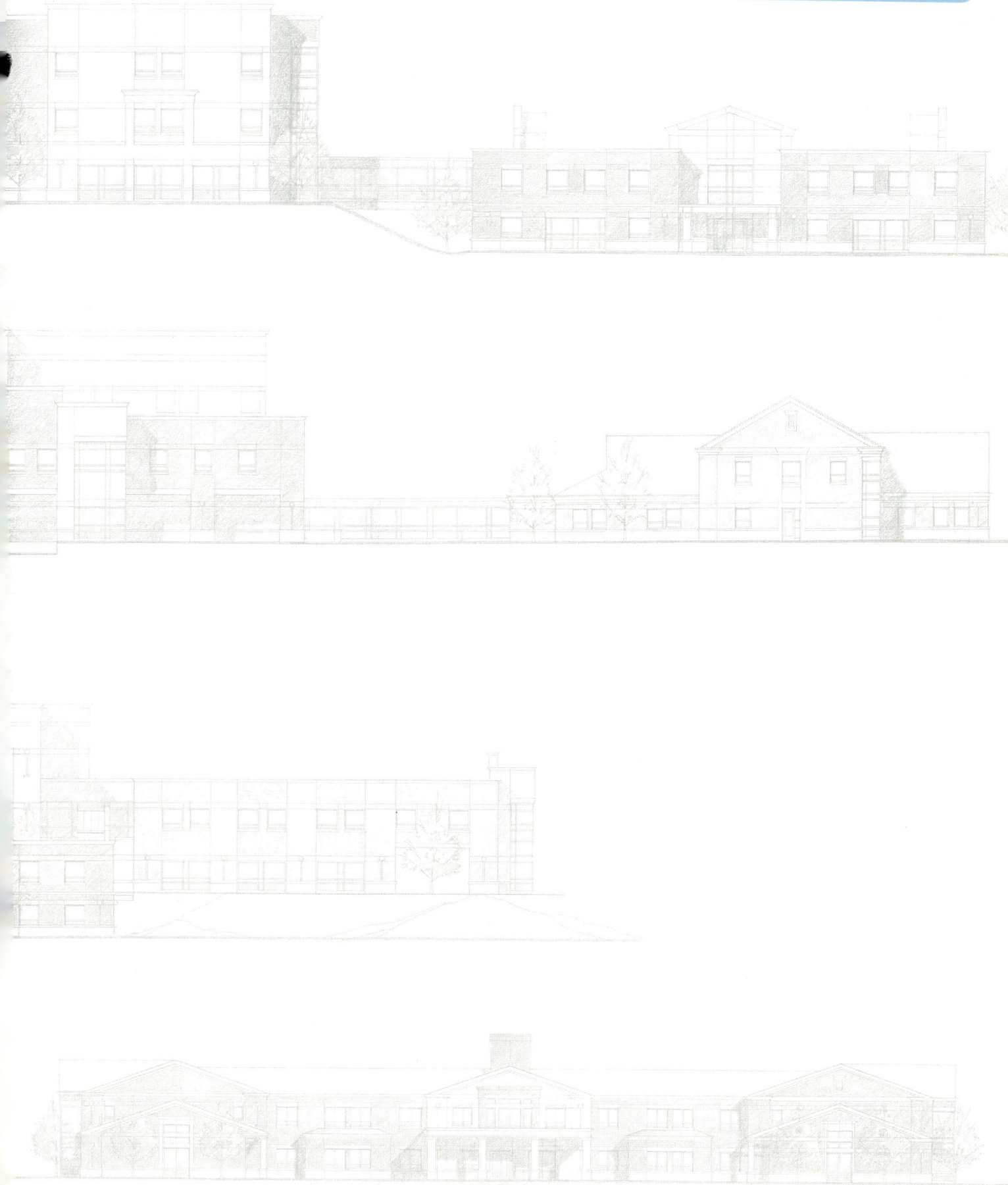

A CENTURY OF CARING

ALLIANCE COMMUNITY HOSPITAL

∽

COMPILED BY
DR. KELLY LOWE

Copyright © May 2002 Alliance Community Hospital

All rights reserved. No portion of this book may be reproduced by any means, electronic or mechanical, including photocopying, recording, or by any information storage retrieval system, without the written permission of the copyright's owner, except for the inclusion of brief quotations for review.

ISBN 0-9718158-0-1

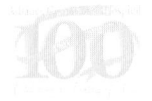

Ted Abel of TA Creative Design created the Centennial logo and provided various scanned photos.

2673 TR 421
Sugarcreek, OH 44681

Carlisle Printing
WALNUT CREEK

Dedication

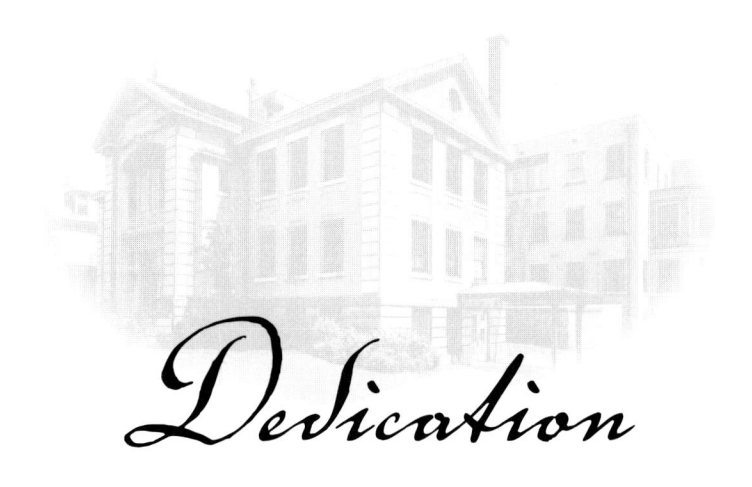

To all those

who served

our community

the first hundred years...

...to all those

carrying forward

our dream and making it

a reality.

Acknowledgments

SEVERAL PEOPLE have been of extraordinary assistance during the writing of this project: Karen Vrabec and Larry Halm have been very helpful in getting me access to the hospital's archives and current staff. My two research assistants, Nicole Matthews and Megan Dooling, both of Mount Union College, now know more about the first fifty years of Alliance history than they ever thought they would. Robert Garland, Cheryl Paine, and the staff of the Mount Union College Library were very gracious as they let me essentially live in the Historical room and the Microfilm area during the summer of 2000. Several members of the Alliance community graciously gave pictures or shared personal memories with me. These include Richard Curtis, Kenneth Swartz, Barbara Ossler, and Craig Bara. Stan Jonas, the current CEO of Alliance Community Hospital, took valuable time with me on a very rainy day in late July, 2001. Much of what Mr. Jonas and I discussed has not found its way into the final manuscript, but his excellent and insightful discussion of the changes the hospital has undergone in the last ten years and the challenges it faces in the next ten informs much of the last chapter. Finally, my wife, Lori Van Houten, and our daughter, Evangeline, have spent the last eighteen months listening to stories about the hospital and haven't yet told me to leave. Thanks.

Contents

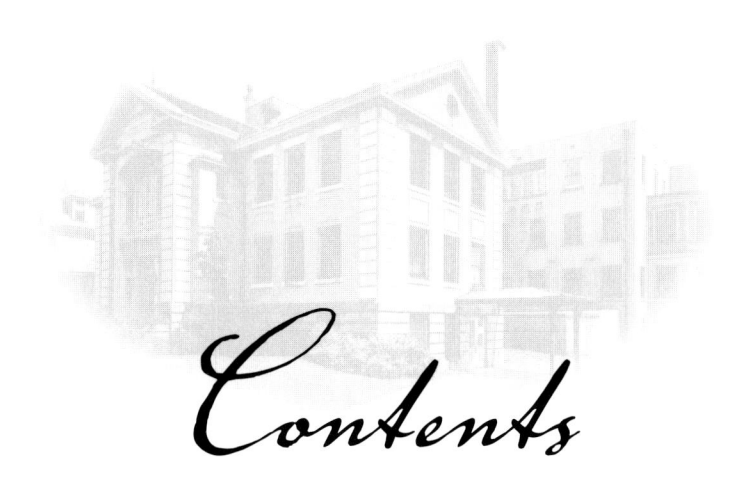

INTRODUCTION 1

FOUNDING: 1900–1910 7

1910–1920 17

1920–1930 27

1930–1940 43

1940–PRESENT 55

THE FUTURE 93

PHOTO GALLERY 101

APPENDIX 125

A CENTURY OF CARING

Introduction

Introduction

It is easy, in the writing of any sort of history, to overestimate the influence of one person on the development of an institution. Often historians want to see the great men and women of our collective historical past as giants upon whose shoulders we all stand. However attractive this method of writing history might be, it is important to resist the idea that any one person should receive a share of credit disproportionate to their contribution.

The Alliance Community Hospital is just that—a *community* hospital—a hospital by, for, and about the community of Alliance. And while there have been individuals who have played significant roles in the development of the hospital from its origins as The Reformed Deaconess Home and Hospital Association to its present incarnation as Alliance Community Hospital, the hospital is truly part of the city of Alliance.

According to the original constitution of the Reformed Deaconess Home, the mission of the hospital and its employees upon founding, was "…to care for the sick whether physically or spiritually, and to engage in such other forms of charitable and benevolent work which may commend themselves to the association".[1] Which, of course, the hospital has managed to do, through war, depression, and near continuous debate over the quality of local drinking water[2], for 100 years – one need not look much further than the meningitis scare of 2001 to see that the hospital takes its community mission very seriously.

A few words about the writing of this history: I have relied, with a few small exceptions, (as the reader will no doubt gather) almost exclusively on the reporting from the *Alliance Review* as well as (in later years) the hospital's *Annual Reports*. I have done this for a few reasons: first, the hospital's archives are nonexistent until after World War II. In the hospital's archives are an annual report from 1902, some information about an early graduating class from the nursing school, and two uncredited (and largely incomplete) histories of the hospital. I used these histories as a guide, but they were, in general, inconsistent, especially in terms of the spelling of names and the accuracy of key dates.

Second, because of the size of Alliance and the importance of the hospital within the community, I felt fairly certain that any and all developments of the hospital would be considered "news". I wasn't disappointed. As my research assistants and I researched the hospital's origins, we looked at every issue of the *Alliance Review* (including the *Weekly Review* and something called the *Review & Leader*) from 1899 to 1940, and found that, with very few exceptions, any information about the hospital was front-page, above-the-fold news.

I have tried to carefully cite all of the *Review* articles that I used in one of two ways: either in the text of the work itself or in a footnote (in the interest of saving space, I haven't done both). It is my hope that if someone else wishes to continue this work (or use it as the basis for some other project) they will find the documentation helpful. Towards the end of this work, as I began to rely more on the information in the hospital's archives and as the deadline pressure began to mount, I found that many of the articles in the carefully kept scrapbooks at the hospital had been cut out of the *Review* without a date. I have tried, to the best of my ability given the schedule I was keeping, to place the articles in historical context to give the reader some idea of what was happening when.

A second thing readers might notice is that after World War II, the coverage of the hospital's growth is done on a less systematic/ year-by-year basis. This was done for a very specific reason: I tend to feel that "history" is something that shouldn't be written until well after the fact – as this project got closer to the time of the writing of the text I felt that the project would be best served by listing the various accomplishments and changes that the hospital has gone through. For instance, much of the documentation available about recent developments with the hospital lists new equipment that the hospital has bought, or new services it has introduced – *there is no real way to evaluate which of these additions will be historically significant* (in the way the purchase of the first X-ray machine undoubtedly was).

There are some things I wish I could have covered more completely in this history, the foremost being the history of the nursing school and the relationship between the nurses and the hospital. The hospital, which started as a Deaconess home and nurses' academy, dropped the nursing school in the late 1940's and I would have liked to have known more about why. For all of the interest in the hospital that was shown by the *Review*, the nursing school was virtually ignored by the newspaper until it was time to tear it down (and even then most of the outrage was about tearing down the historic building that housed the nursing home and not about the loss of the nursing school *per se*). I would have liked to have known more about the nurses' strike in 1976 and the history of women doctors at the hospital.

Several readers of this book while still in manuscript form commented that there was little or no information about the Auxiliary, the Doctors' Wives (who used to throw a major benefit every year), and the Foundation. It would be an interesting project, albeit one that this history is not set up to tackle, to look specifically at the place that women have had at the hospital, as employees and as a very significant support system.[3]

The Foundation is a special case. Its importance to the hospital is unquestioned. The main reason it is absent from this history (beyond some information about its origins) is that it is difficult to determine, historically, what sort of place the Foundation plays (or will play) in regards to the history of the hospital. Perhaps when the 150th anniversary rolls around, the Foundation's role will be given some much needed historical perspective.

One more note: this history is not an objective study of the hospital's social/cultural/political place in the Alliance community—it is a celebratory and documentary history of the hospital's first 100 years. There were, as I researched the history, many voices who have spoken out about various elements of the hospital's progress (especially, though not limited to, the most recent expansion of the hospital along College Avenue). I have, for the most part, left out the criticism (much of which saw the light of day in the form of letters to the editor in the *Alliance Review*). In only one instance do I include much criticism: during the attempts to raise money for an addition in the early fifties and the concurrent move to change the hospital's administration from city owned and run to an independent board of trustees, there was a heated battle over the proposals that caused at least one man to run for mayor on the single issue of defeating the change in administration and another to take out what must have been thousands of dollars worth of paid advertisements in the *Review* against the changes. I found this drama too rich to ignore.

A CENTURY OF CARING

Founding: 1900–1910

Founding: 1900–1910

History shows us that we owe the origin of hospitals, not to medical science, but to religion. It need not astonish us to learn that hospitals (houses for the sick) were known in ante-Christian times. That they were not found with the cultured Greeks and Romans, but with the Buddhists, is proof that they are not the result of culture and civilization, but of religion.[4]

It is a great understatement to say that America was different at the dawn of the 20th century than it is now at the dawn of the 21st. In the year 1900, William McKinley, of Canton, Ohio, was thinking about re-election (he would win the Presidency that November, in a close race with William Jennings Bryan). Oklahoma, New Mexico, Arizona, Alaska, and Hawaii were still not states. Melville Fuller was the Chief Justice of the Supreme Court of the United States. There were, in 1900, six cities in the United States that were as big as London and Paris. Per capita income was $450 per year, while the richest 2% of the country owned roughly 60% of its wealth. The industrial base of the country was organized around railroads, iron and steel, meatpacking, milling, tobacco, and petroleum.

Like much of the progress that occurred at

J. H. TRESSEL, M. D.

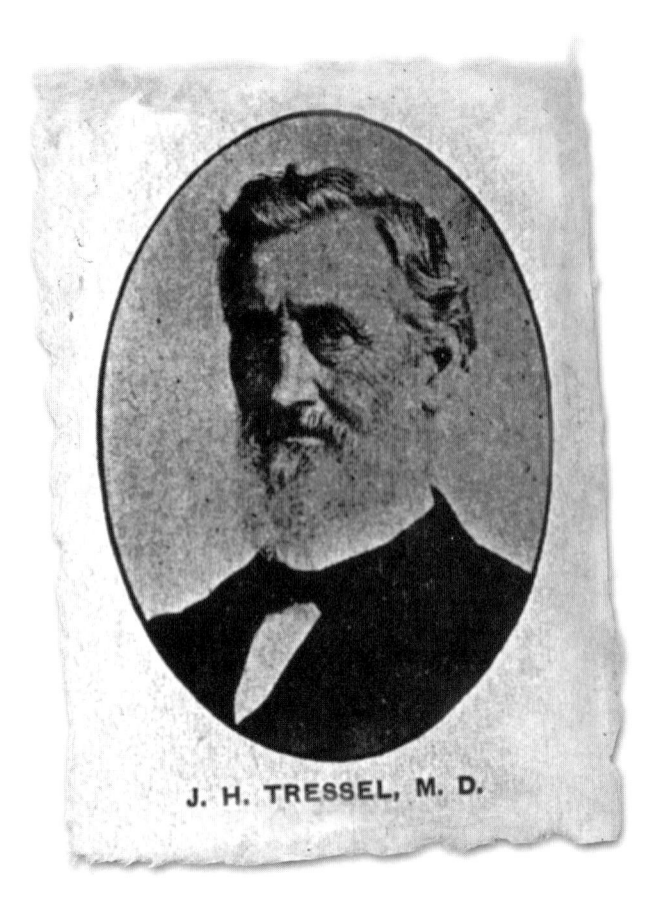

the beginning of the twentieth century, the story of the Alliance Community Hospital begins with a church. In the year 1900, Dr. J.H. Tressel, a local physician, suggested to the Reverend H. E. Kilmer of the Immanuel Reformed Church of Alliance that a hospital was needed. By all accounts, the Reverend Kilmer was an enthusiastic man, and he set about trying to organize the hospital, raise funds, and find a staff. The June 29, 1900 edition of the *Alliance Daily Review* reports that

> Such an institution would not only receive a great number of injured people for surgical operation and treatment during each year but many sick people would be taken to the hospital that they might have the benefit of hospital care, hospital quietude and the proper environment.[5]

On January 18, 1900, Kilmer, Tressel, and others[6] came together to constitute the Reformed Deaconess Home and Hospital Association with the purpose of having both a hospital and a Deaconess training facility.[7] In the constitution for the Reformed Deaconess Home was the mission "...to care for the sick whether physically or spiritually, and to engage in such other forms of charitable and benevolent work which may commend themselves to the association".[8] The Association was incorporated under the laws of the State of Ohio on April 12, 1900.[9]

Eight months later, on December 8, 1900, the Hospital Association took possession of the Whitacre house, which was located on the corner of Arch and College Streets. The Hospital Association paid $4000 for the house, raised mainly through small donations. For the most part there was "universal encouragement" for the building of the hospital, though there was some concern by the neighbors that the hospital would be "something of a pest house." The hospital assured its neighbors that "no contagious diseases will be admitted and that it [the hospital] will be in all respects attractive."[10]

The Reverend Kilmer's mother-in-law, Mrs.

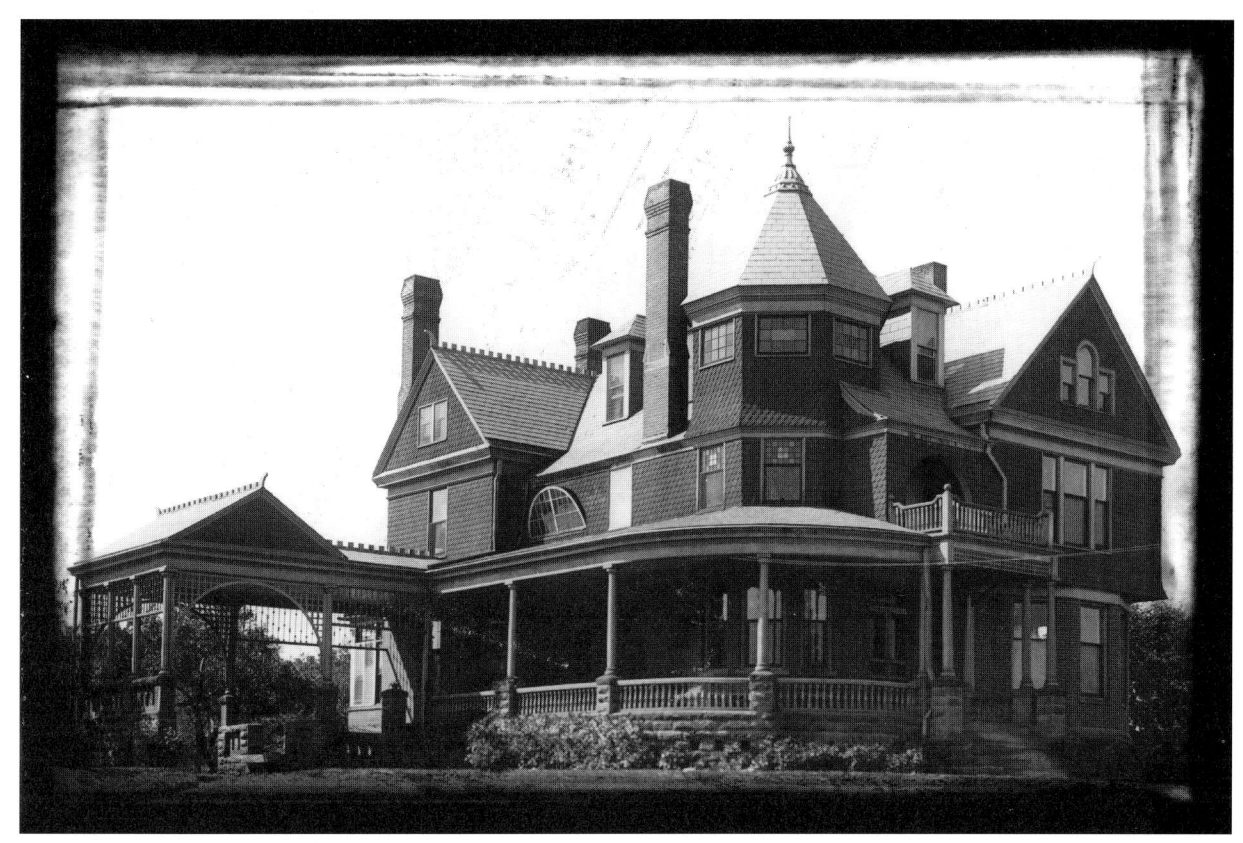

[Whitacre Home in 1902]

M.E. Whitmore, moved into the house immediately upon purchase in order to "protect the property" and to oversee the refurbishing of the property.[11] The first year was, according to Mrs. Whitmore's diary, one of "hard toil, sacrifice, and many great trials."

On January 2, 1901, Mrs. Rose Chenot, of Louisville, OH, joined Mrs. Whitmore in the Whitacre house to help refurbish it. This was the same day that the plumbers and electricians started working to convert the home from a residence to a hospital.

The early medical organization of the hospital was simple: Dr. Tressel was the natural and obvious choice as chief of staff. Miss Margaret Ubert of Baltimore was the first head nurse and acting matron. She was followed in quick succession by Miss Lula Henneberger of Hagerstown, MD, and Miss Reinecke of Nazareth, PA. Early nurses in the Deaconess system studied Bible Exposition, Christian Doctrine, Christian Worship, Church History, Evidences, Catechesis, the Deaconate, German and English Grammar, Principles and Method, Nursing and Household Economy, Hygiene, Anatomy, and Materia Medica.[12]

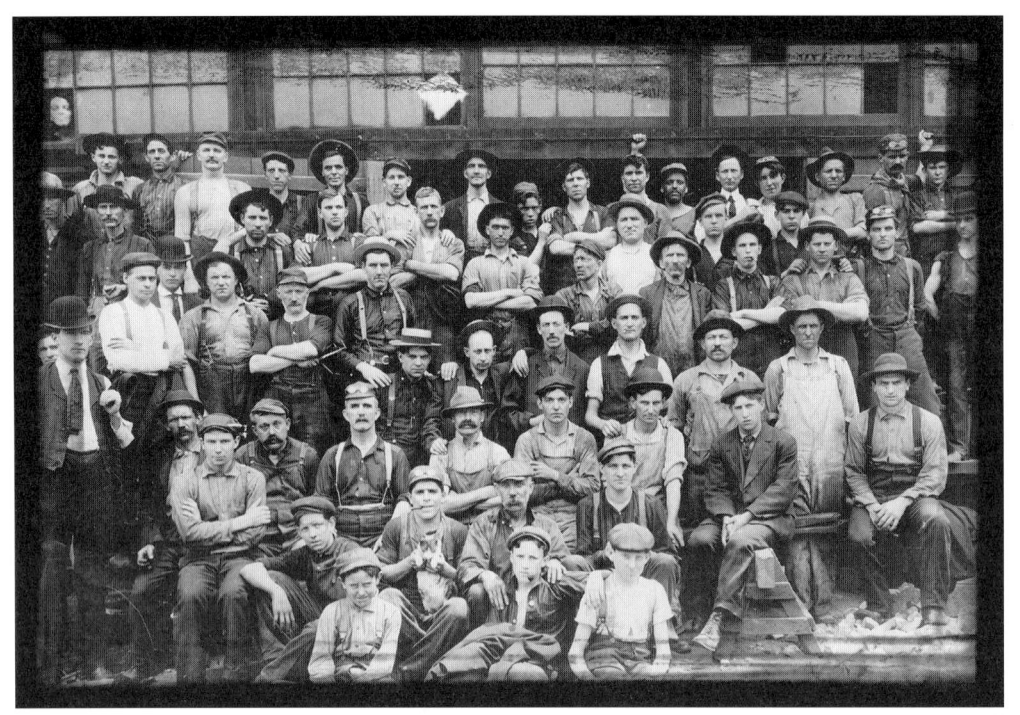

[ALLIANCE FACTORY WORKERS IN 1910]

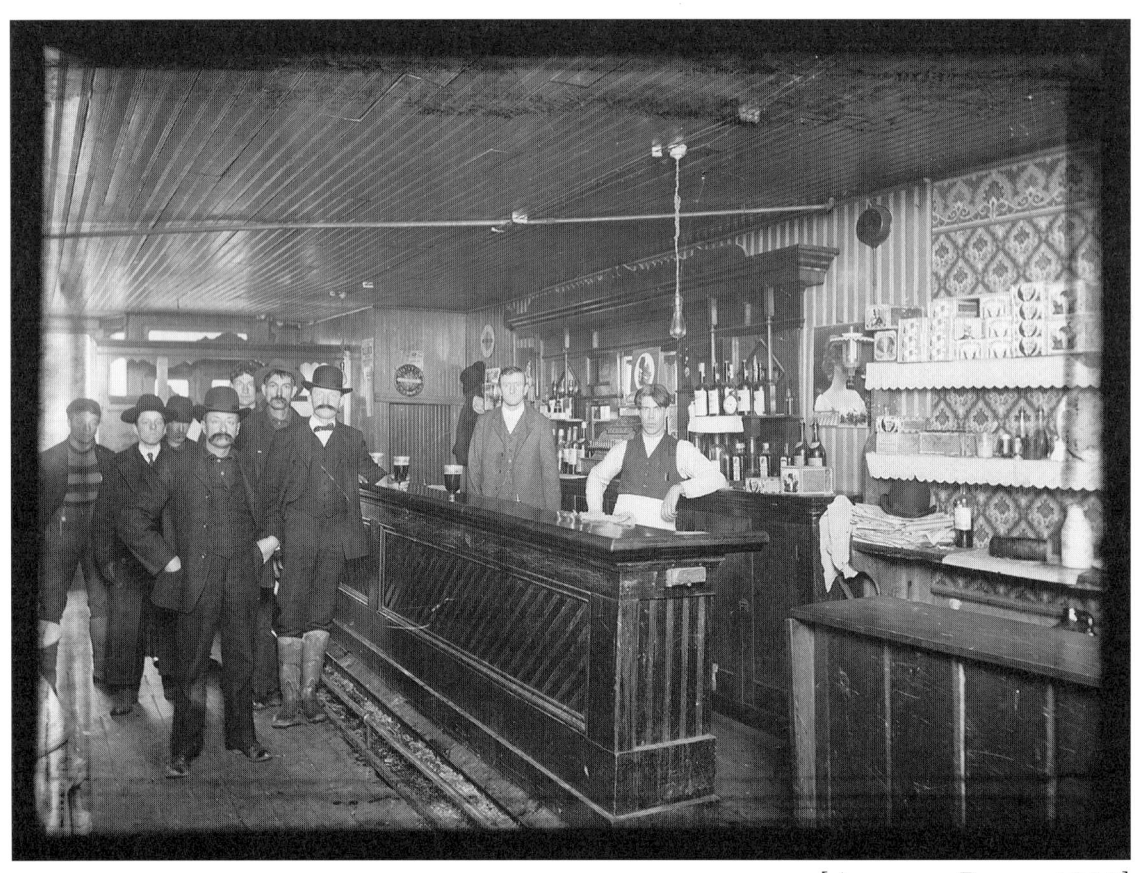

[ALLIANCE BAR IN 1903]

The surgical staff was made up of Doctors P.C. Ramsey, J.A. Douglas, George Haffert, and William Merchant. The medical staff included Doctors C.M. Hoover, P.W. Welker, D.M. Johnson, and J.A. Roach.

The Deaconess Home was only the second hospital in Stark County (Aultman Hospital in Canton had been founded eight years earlier by Katherine Aultman and Elizabeth Harter); facilities at its inception were somewhat limited: twenty beds with cornhusk mattresses. There were also rooms for nurses and housekeepers.[13]

An interesting piece of trivia about the early hospital is that, according to historian C. Golder, the Reformed Deaconess Home and Hospital may well have been the first Deaconess home to operate under the auspices of the Reformed Church.[14] Golder writes that "The first English Deaconess Institute of this denomination [Reformed Church (English-speaking) of the United States] was established by a few of its members at Alliance, O."[15]

The early operation of the hospital was organized by the aforementioned Hospital Association. According to the *Alliance Daily Review*,

> *Members of the [Hospital] association may be either annual or life members. Any person may become an annual member by contributing at least two dollars annually. Any person may become a life member who shall contribute $25 at one time.*[16]

In keeping with the Christian and charitable mission of the hospital,

> *Those who are able to pay for the accommodations are expected to do so according to a fixed scale of prices. Those unable to pay will be cared for so long as the resources of the association will possibly permit.*[17]

By 1906, the hospital was enough a part of Alliance that the *Daily Review* was able to write

[GRADE 4 · NORTH PARK]

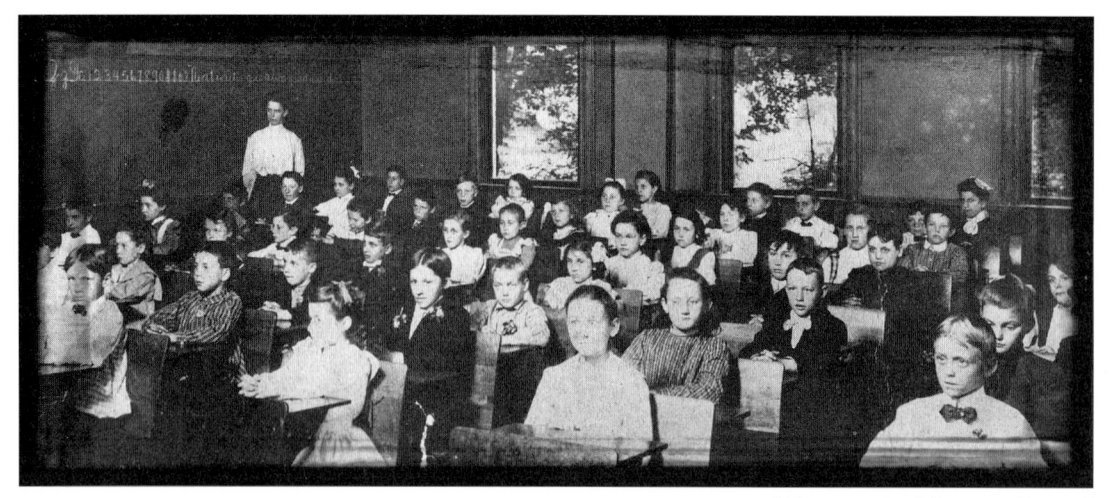

that "The hospital proves a boon of inestimable value to the city and surrounding towns."

The second big event that occurred during the hospital's early, formative years was the founding of the nursing school in 1903. Due to two fires at the hospital (in 1909 and 1911), much of the information about the nursing school has been lost or destroyed. According to the hospital's records, the nursing school was run by the doctors (who taught the classes). The nurses-in-training were given a five- to eight-dollar allowance each month as well as room, board, and laundry (uniforms, which were to be worn at all times, were to be procured at the trainee's own expense). The nursing program, according to an early application, was a three-year program.

According to the Second *Annual Report* (1902), the hospital, by 1903, was a thriving concern. Some interesting figures from the report:

· *Number of patients from January 1, 1902 to January 1, 1903: 151*
· *Number of days of hospital service: 2603*
· *Dismissed recovered: 96*
· *Dismissed improved: 25*
· *Dismissed unimproved: 13*
· *Deaths (six of whom were hopeless when admitted): 10*

By the end of its first decade, the hospital was in sound financial shape. It was an obviously important part of the community, and its doctors and nurses were graciously giving back to Alliance through their ministrations to the poor.

There is some question as to when the Reformed Deaconess Home and Hospital became Alliance City Hospital. According to the hospital's records, it was in 1912, but already, by 1906, the *Alliance Daily Review* is writing about the "Alliance City Hospital", and the name appears to have been changed officially and for good in 1908.[18]

Regardless of when and why, the name was changed because the Reformed Church was having a great deal of difficulty running the institution, and they needed the city's help in managing and funding the hospital. According to the May 29, 1906 issue of the *Daily Review*, "Few hospitals anywhere pay all expenses from the receipts of the patients." This was a problem because expenses had quickly surpassed revenues, and while the new City Hospital fully intended to maintain its charity mission, the need to increase the medical staff's (both doctors and nurses) salaries was an overwhelming concern. The *Daily Review* paints a pretty bleak picture:

> The head nurse, with all the responsibility resting upon her, receives less than she could command as a private nurse. … If the hospital is allowed to close, who will have the courage and set about the task to re-establish it? Unless help is secured such must be the result. The members of the board are all business or professional men who can illy afford to give the time necessary for the proper management of the hospital, but they give it cheerfully and gratis. Their service is not only without compensation, but often carries with it censure, because the ideas of all cannot be carried out in the conduct of the institution.[19]

The first move towards fiscal responsibility seems to have been taken in 1908 with the revision of the hospital's constitution and a move towards a more nonsectarian mission. According to the January 11, 1908 edition of the *Review*, a new board of fifteen directors was chosen.

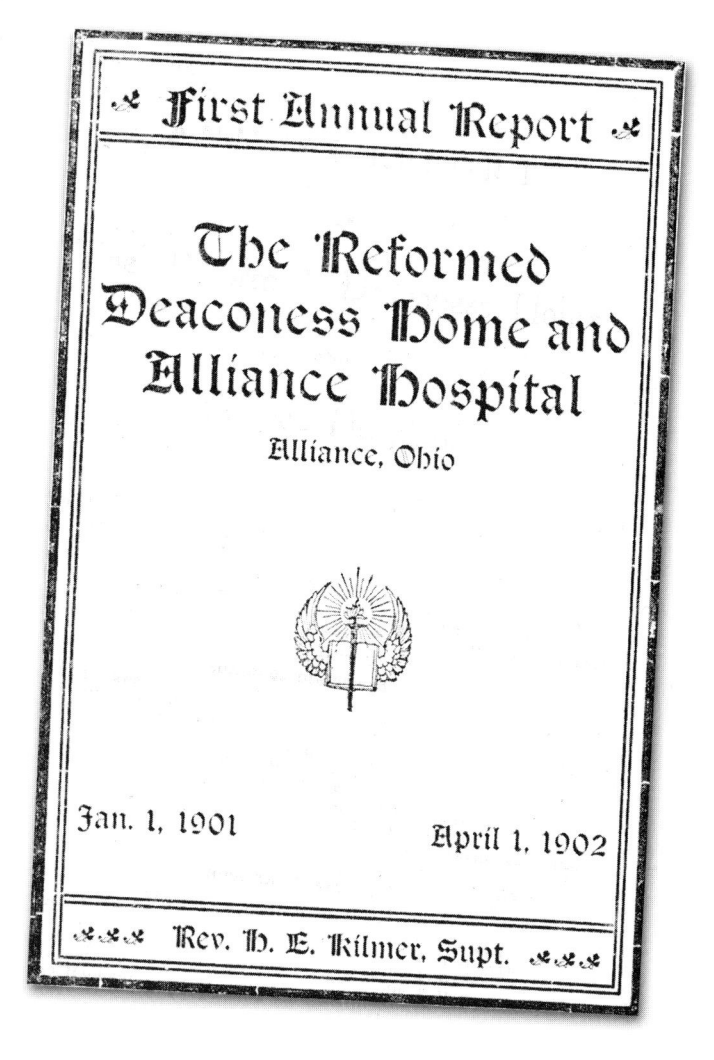

Some highlights of the new constitution:

ARTICLE 1: The name of the corporation shall be the Alliance City Hospital Association.

ARTICLE 2: Object:
- Sec. 1: to maintain a modern hospital conducted on nonsectarian principles.
- Sec. 2: to care for the sick and injured.
- Sec. 3: to maintain a nurses' training school and grant nursing diplomas.
- Sec. 4: dispense gratuitously, hospital service, to deserving poor and unfortunate, otherwise not provided for.

ARTICLE 3: Membership:
- Sec. 1: shall consist of lifetime and annual members.
- Sec. 2: anyone who contributes $25 will be a lifetime member.
- Sec. 3: $2 contribution will make for an annual member (from the day of contribution).
- Sec. 4: membership is not transferable.
- Sec. 5: each member gets one vote.
- Sec. 6: practicing physicians can be members of association, but may not be members of the board of directors.

ARTICLE 4: Management

ARTICLE 5: Officers

ARTICLE 6: Annual meeting

ARTICLE 7: Superintendent

ARTICLE 8: Hospital Staff

ARTICLE 9: Benefits of the Hospital
- Sec. 1: the hospital shall be for the sick and injured. Wards and private rooms shall be open to all. No national or denominational lines should be recognized.
- Sec. 2: Those who are capable of paying should continue to do so by offered arrangements.

ARTICLE 10: By-laws

ARTICLE 11: Amendment.

The original members of this board were: Norman C. Fetters, A.G. Reeves, B.F. Weybrecht, John Eyer, Wm. Lindesmith, H.I. Allen, W.I. Murphy, O.F. Transug, G.W. Shem, Frank Cassaday, H.C. Koehler, W.H. Ramsey, J.H. Lloyd, J.S. Spring, and G.H. Souder.

According to the same article in the *Alliance Review*, the first order of business, which would consume the board throughout the next decade, was the need for expansion.

A CENTURY OF CARING

1910–1920

1910—1920

By all accounts, the years 1910-1920 were turbulent: for America, for Alliance, and for the hospital. During the same time that the hospital was changing ownership and more than doubling its size, Alliance was worrying about the quality of its water, the infiltration of the crime gang known as the "black hand" into the city, the abusive treatment of the residents of the Fairmount home for boys, the merger of Mount Union and Scio colleges, and whether to build electric streetlights on Main Street. The world saw the Titanic sink, Pancho Villa run rampant in Mexico and Texas, the bizarrely comical election of 1912 (remember the Bull-Moose party?) and, of course, the devastating war in Europe.[20]

Like many charitable organizations, the Deaconess Home struggled during its early years to balance charity with its mission to sustain itself as a business. In other words, it was a victim of its own success—the hospital had quickly outgrown the Whitacre property and was plagued by debts and desperately in need of a new physical plant.

With this in mind, it was decided in 1912 to change the name of the Hospital Association to the Alliance City Hospital Association and to start thinking about the place of the hospital within the city's infrastructure. The April 26, 1912 edition of the Alliance *Weekly Review* reports that there were "Plans for a Proposed New Alliance Hospital." The story continues:

> *There are now 20 patients in the hospital, nearly all of whom are what is denominated operating or emergency patients and to accommodate all of these, cots have been placed in the hospital hall and in single rooms as many as 3 beds have been placed.*

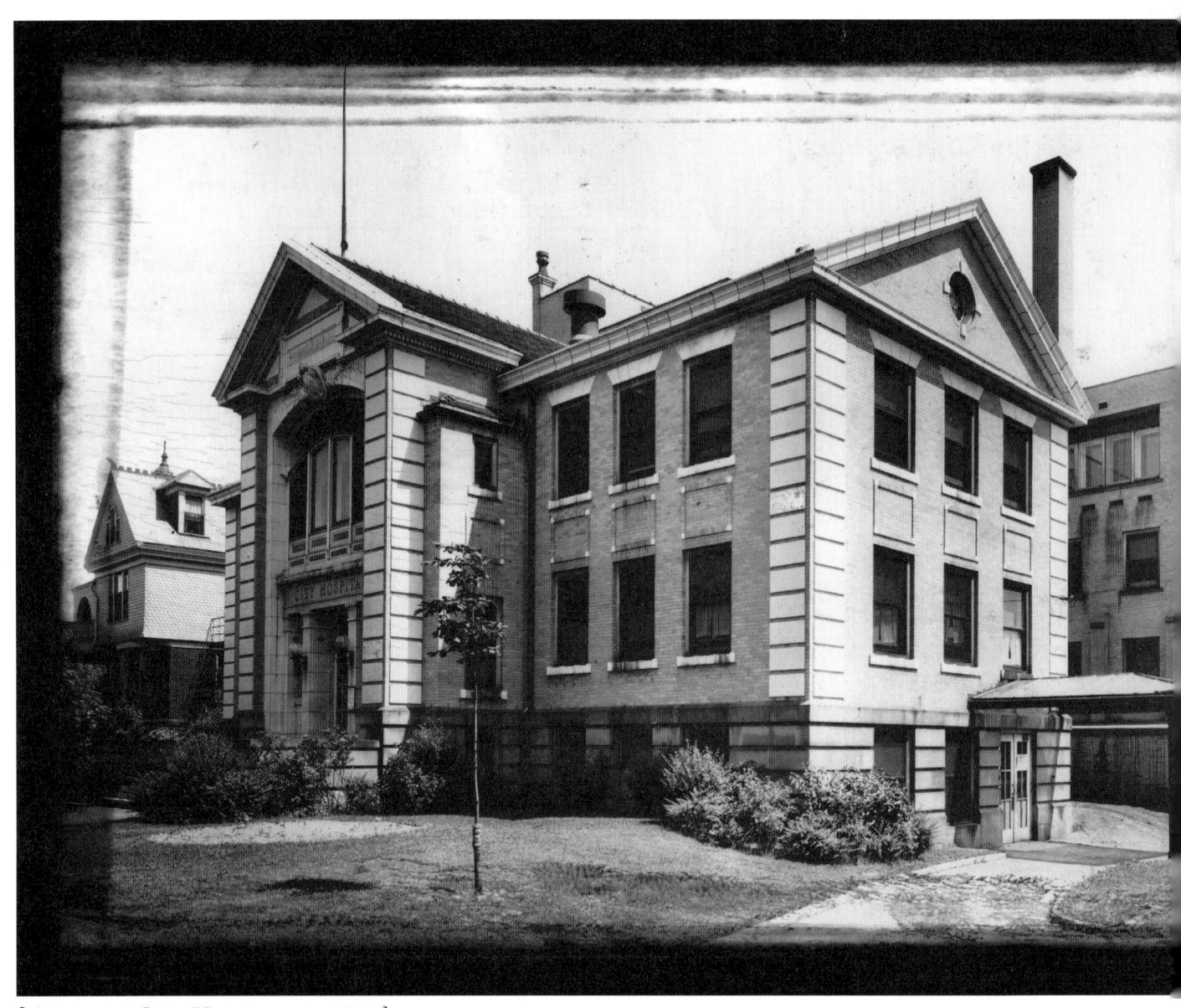

[ALLIANCE CITY HOSPITAL IN 1917]

... The need for a great hospital for the city has never been greater.

The story lists C.C. and A.C. Thayer, of New Castle, PA as the architects (they would, however, be replaced by a firm out of Cleveland when the hospital commission actually began building the new hospital).

The desire of the hospital board was to have a facility that could house 50 patients at a time. The design would be three stories high with a fireproof basement. There would be men's and women's operating rooms, "widely separated" from one another. It was estimated that the hospital would cost $1,000 per room to build, and that room charges would be on a sliding scale from $30 per room per week to $7, with charitable cases paid for by the hospital.

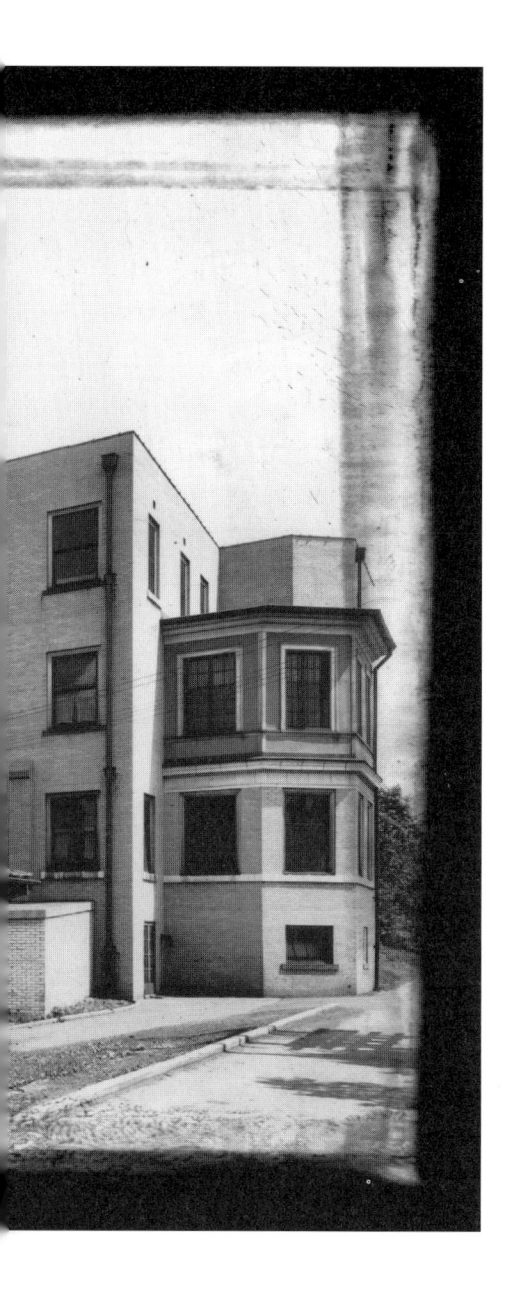

On Tuesday, November 18, 1913, The *Weekly Review* reported that the city was seeking a $50,000 bond ordinance, proposed by Mr. Voss, for the building of the new hospital, and a second ordinance for the "appropriation of land." The bond issues were passed on December 2, 1913.

The business of the hospital went on as usual during this time. The *Weekly Review* reported that, on December 3, 1913, the hospital received donations from local schoolchildren, including "243 quarts of fruit, vegetables, soap, sugar, flour, and biscuits."

After the name change and the passage of the bond issue, the board moved to change the very structure of the hospital, and in late 1913 it was decided to deed the hospital to the city, with the city taking over the administration of the hospital. The December 9, 1913 issue of the *Alliance Review* reports that a Mr. Farmer proposed a plan to purchase the present hospital property and to lease the property back to the hospital board for a minimum of twenty-five years. While, in general, city council seemed to favor the move (which would eventually make the mayor and members of the city council members of the city hospital board), it did not pass through council as swiftly as members of the hospital board hoped it would. There were endless meetings between the hospital board and the city council. The election of a new mayor and city council, who promptly came in and attempted to rewrite most of the already agreed upon transfer agreement, delayed the progress considerably.

The January 17, 1914 issue of the *Alliance Review* reports that the Alliance City Hospital Association had formally arranged for the city to take charge of the hospital. According to the terms of the agreement, the city would take over all of the property/real estate owned by the hospital board "provided the city in return would obligate itself to erect a modern hospital." However, the January 27 issue of the *Review* reports that city council and the hospital board were "almost deadlocked" on the terms of agreement, which had mainly to do with how much land the city would get from the hospital.

A CENTURY OF CARING   *1910—1920* · 21

Finally, on February 16, 1914, the city council accepted the hospital property. Thus the city took over the hospital on the condition that it would provide the land for a new, larger facility. On June 2 of the same year, city council accepted the recommendation of the hospital commission to hire Willard Hirsh of Cleveland to design and build the hospital. Hirsh would do so for a payment of 6% of the cost of the building.[21] Soon after, a building committee was appointed, chaired by Mr. C. M. Hoover; the aforementioned $50,000 bond issue was approved by the voters of the city of Alliance; and the construction of the hospital began.

According to one unattributed history of the hospital, the fundraising and subsequent construction of the new hospital was not an easy task. A newly organized women's auxiliary worked countless hours organizing and fundraising for the new physical plant, some going so far as to buy lots for the new site.[22]

By September of 1916 the improved physical plant was complete. The *Daily Review* noted that the "City Hospital [is] to be Turned Over Thursday." The building commission, which was responsible for overseeing the building of the physical plant, turned the building over to the city to furnish. The city, by this point, was nervous because there was not enough money left to furnish the hospital the way it needed to be. The *Review* states that there was enough money left for "appointments" in the operating rooms, private rooms, and wards, but that the overall operation of the hospital would be delayed and when the hospital did open it would cost, on average, 8-9 times more to run than did the "old" hospital.[23]

The lack of funds (because the city used most of the equipment money on the building itself) led to a city-wide fund drive. The mayor of Alliance asked "churches, benevolent societies, and organizations such as lodges and private individuals" for contributions. The mayor hoped that "some benevolent individuals may be induced to furnish a room on the endowment plan."[24]

Before the hospital could be completely furnished, however, tragedy struck. The September 29 edition of the *Alliance Daily Review and Leader* reported

> *that immediate action should be taken to rush the city hospital building to completion or at least so that a portion can be used was most vividly exemplified Friday afternoon when an injured man lay in an ambulance for nearly an hour and a half awaiting some arrangements for being placed in a bed.*

The man was first treated in the mayor's office and then transferred, at city expense, to a hospital in Canton. The mayor launched an immediate investigation, citing the fact that it had been "over two years since the bond [for the new physical plant] was approved."[25]

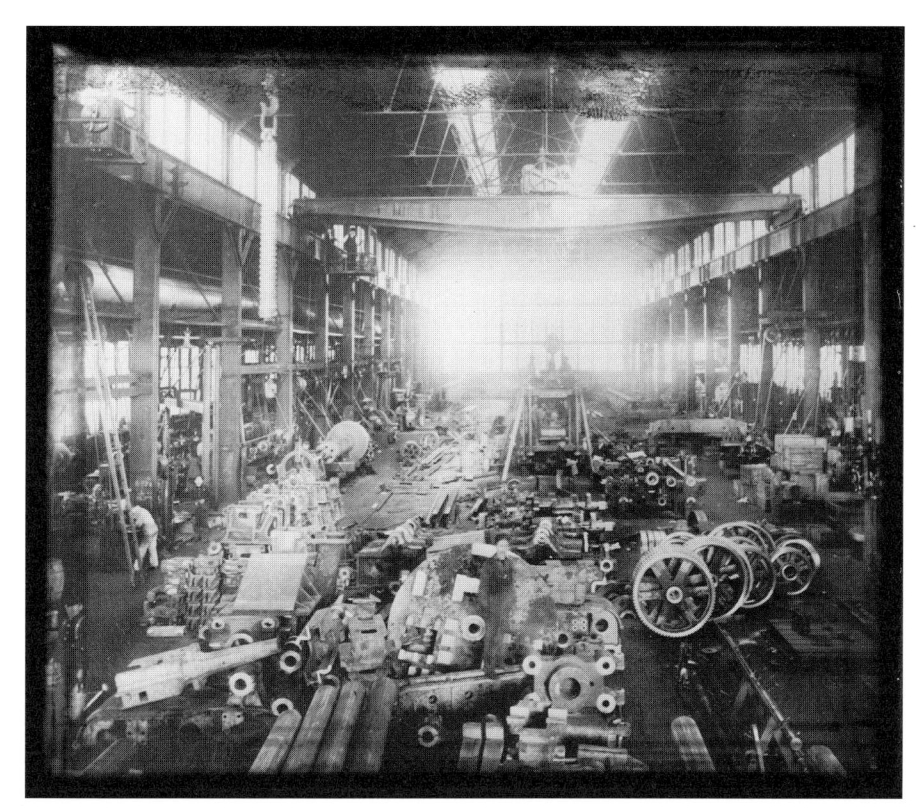

[ALLIANCE FACTORY IN 1913]

tended the grand opening ceremonies. The *Alliance Review and Leader* reported, in its January 2, 1917 edition, that

The formal opening of the new city hospital for inspection by the public occurred Monday [January 1] afternoon and evening. Cut flowers were the contributed decorations of the interior of the building, giving it a cheerful appearance. During the hours the hospital was open a constant stream of visitors availed themselves of the privilege of seeing a model hospital and were much interested in the style and arrangement of the building and the appliances for use. ... The nurses from the old hospital in neat uniforms, acted as ushers for the visitors. There was no formal program and no speech making.

It was stated today that the new building is now ready and it is more than probable pa-

The upshot of this terrible event was that less than two weeks later the *Review* was reporting that the "Hospital will be furnished at once," as a result of both public and political pressure. The city council voted unanimously to give money to finish and furnish the hospital. At the same time, council voted to give $15,000 to refurbish the old site of the Deaconess home to become the permanent nurses' home.[26]

By late December of 1916, the *Review* was able to report that the new hospital would soon be "thrown open to [the] city." On January 1, 1917, the Alliance City Hospital was formally opened. More than 2,500 citizens at-

[NURSES C. 1920]

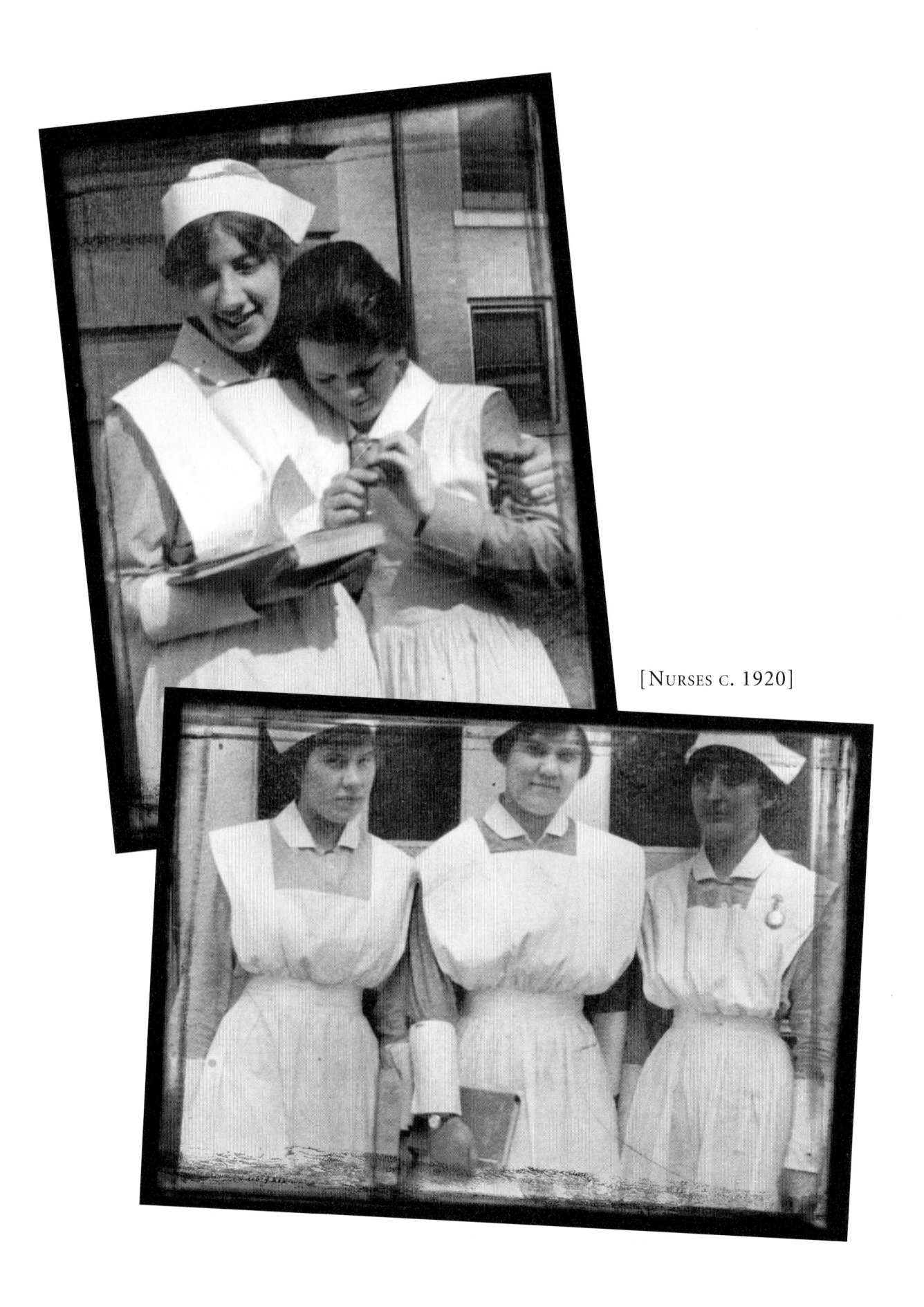

24 · *1910—1920*   A CENTURY OF CARING

tients will be received for this Wednesday. A number of sick have applications waiting to be admitted.

Once the new hospital was up and running, it was business as usual. On January 20th, the *Review* reported that due to "growing pains", the hospital would add five more nurses. The story also reported that in 1916, there were 582 cases at the old hospital.[27]

On February 21, 1917, the City Hospital was declared

> "complete" and ready for business. It was reported that Safety Director J.H. Patton has made a careful computation as regards the cost of operating the hospital and with the sanction of the hospital board has made a scale of prices hoping to make the hospital as self-sustaining as possible.

Patton set the prices as follows: a stay in a ward was priced at $10.50 - $12.50 per week; a semiprivate room was $15.00 per week; a private room was $15.00 - $30.00 per week. "Alliance," wrote the paper, "is proud of her hospital and the privileges it affords should not be abused."[28]

After the excitement of the new building, the hospital settled down to serve the community. News of the hospital stopped being a daily event (in part, no doubt, because of the daily headlines about World War I and its aftermath). Occasionally, however, something interesting, unusual, or special occurred. On November 1, 1917, for instance, the *Review* reported on the front page that twins were born two days apart, one being born at the home of its mother, Mrs. Annie Rampelt, and the other being born at the City Hospital via cesarean section and the "Porro Method." Both mother and babies, it was reported, were doing fine.[29]

All in all, it was a good thing that the hospital was finished when it was. With the advent of World War I and the post-war economic difficulties, several bond issues (for schools, for city hall, for an improved water plant, and for lights on Main Street) were all rejected by the voters in the 1918, 1919, and 1920 elections.

For the hospital, the years 1910-1920 ended on a good, peaceful note. The last mention of the hospital in this decade is in the December 27 edition of the *Review* which reported on the hospital's Christmas party, which included a "large, well-lighted Christmas tree, fruit and candy, and the singing of carols." The tree was donated by the Schaffer-Black Company and was wired by Chief Held and an assistant. Santa Claus was portrayed by Dr. Warren Unger. The physicians of the hospital gave the nurses a "large bookcase" for the nurses' home; the home received several magazine subscriptions as well as "records for the Victrola." Finally, the Junior Mission band of the Friends Church distributed personal Christmas greetings to all 45 patients in the hospital.[30] It was a nice ending to a nice decade.

A CENTURY OF CARING

1920-1930

1920—1930

Like most of America, Alliance in the period 1920-1930 was experiencing unprecedented growth. While America was struggling with coal strikes, marveling at the bravery of the first daredevil pilots, trying to figure out what was going on at Teapot Dome, following the wars in China and Nicaragua, and reading about Bobby Jones's exploits at the British Open, Alliance was worrying about which streets to pave, where to put a bandstand in Silver Park, watching the building of the Mount Union College Stadium, and arguing about whether the country would be "wet" or "dry".

The twenties were relatively peaceful in terms of the development of the City Hospital. There was much discussion of the hospital's place in the community, ending with another addition during the years 1922-23, and an increasing sense of the need for the hospital to give back to the community – increased charity work, outreach, and involvement by staff in city issues became the hallmarks of the hospital.

There is not much mention of the hospital in the public record between the years 1920-1922; in fact, the first mention is a small piece from January 1922, discussing improvements that the hospital needed. The *Review* states that the improvements were on schedule. The primary necessity was to increase the number of beds in the hospital to 115 and to install a new water softener. There was some discussion of the use of public bond money for these improvements, and as we shall see, the hospital used the bond money and a whole lot more in the addition to come."[31]

On February 1, 1922, the *Alliance Review* reported that the "South Wing of City Hospital May Be Completed April 1." According to

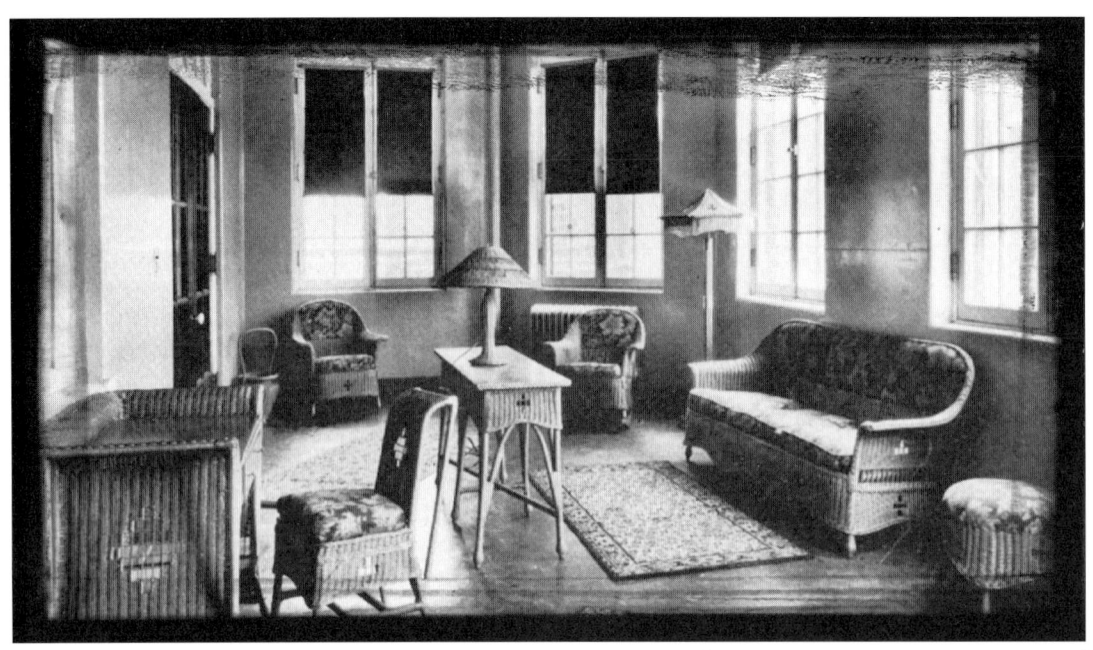

[ACH Waiting Room · 1926]

the story, the plans called for the following:

> *the patients now in the central part of the plant will be moved to the new south wing and the work of raising the building from two to three stories will be begun. No estimate has been placed on when this part of the hospital will be finished.*[32]

Taking a break from the building of the hospital, the local newspaper reports that the Alliance City Hospital was a participant in the second annual National Hospital Day, held on the 102nd birthday of Florence Nightingale. The hospital held an open house so that the community would be able to "come in and see for itself how the sick and the injured of the community are cared for."[33]

Money reared its ugly head again in July 1922 when the administration considered raising the rates to better reflect the costs of doing business in Alliance. The new prices would be: $3 for wards; $4-$5 for private wards; $6 for private rooms (all per day). The new prices were believed to be a "happy medium" between higher rates charged in some institutions and the exceptionally low rates currently charged by Alliance City Hospital.[34]

Economic news was again front and center in September 1922. An article on the front page of the *Review* cited the hospital's operation at an average loss of $438.29 per month (total receipts for August 1922 were $3,872.36).[35]

The relationship between the hospital and the city became quite contentious in October 1922. On Monday, October 16, city council expressed a desire for several changes in the administration of the hospital. These changes included:

30 · 1920—1930   A CENTURY OF CARING

1. That council turn over the buying of all food supplies to the safety director or his designee;
2. That council appoint a visiting committee made up of at least three members of council for the purpose of making a minimum of one inspection a month and that a written report be filed with council and read at the first meeting in the month following. The council would hear and investigate reports from persons who were in any way dissatisfied with their care and treatment while at the hospital;
3. This committee would include the mayor and the safety director as ex officio members;
4. Council formulate a system of rules for the admission of patients from the standpoint of their financial capacity;
5. A plan would be drawn up for a more systematic method of collecting accounts.[36]

These proposed changes in the administration of the hospital by the city led to some interesting discussions in city council. A characteristic headline from October of 1922: "Hospital is Warm Center of Debate at Solons' Meet."

According to the *Review*, an outraged city councilman, Mr. Ryan, spoke at length against the hospital, citing gross "mismanagement," especially in terms of the nursing school. Apparently, the nurses were required by the state to have more education than Mr. Ryan felt was necessary (the nurses needed more laboratory time than they were currently getting). A proposal was before the council requesting funds so the nurses could use some of Mount Union College's laboratory facilities. Ryan, not finding success in his attacks on the hospital management, moved quickly to attack the nurses themselves, complaining that they didn't do their work and were wasting taxpayer money. Ryan was roundly condemned for this statement. Ryan finally ended with an *ad hominem* attack on the management of the hospital, claiming that they were betraying their roots as a charitable organization by not treating those who could not afford to pay. Safety Director Shaw, Councilman Trott, and others roundly refuted Mr. Ryan who then called for adjournment.[37]

The city was learning that running a hospital was difficult, especially in the public eye.

Perhaps one reason for this increased scrutiny of the hospital's management was the increasing need for expansion. The October 5, 1922 issue of the *Review* reports that the hospital had asked the city for an additional $34,000 in bond money to complete an addition that would increase the number of beds in the hospital from sixty to 120 (one bed for every 208 citizens of the city of Alliance).

A few days later the legislation for the bond was passed by city council. The *Review* reported that by "a unanimous vote" the council "enacted the necessary legislation to provide the funds that will enable the city hospital commission to proceed with the furnishing and equipping of the institution and to build a modern laundry."[38] As part of the legislation, a "visiting committee" of three was formed to investigate any and all complaints about the hospital. The committee was made up of three members of city council as well as the mayor and the safety director.

In December 1922, the superintendent of the hospital, Mrs. Charlotte Frye, resigned after five years of service. She had been appointed by the safety director at the time, Mr. Patton, and was praised upon her exit as being responsible for turning the hospital (and especially the nursing school) into one of the best in the country. Some of her accomplishments included helping the hospital to gain certification by the state medical board, improving the classrooms as well as forging relationships with Mount Union College and Cleveland City Hospital (for training the nursing school couldn't do on its own). Mrs. Frye also helped to organize the maternity ward, especially the nursery. She is also given credit for being a driving force for the addition to the hospital's physical plant that was nearly complete. In perhaps the ultimate tribute, the *Alliance Review* wrote that "Mrs. Charlotte Frye has left our city better than she found it."[39]

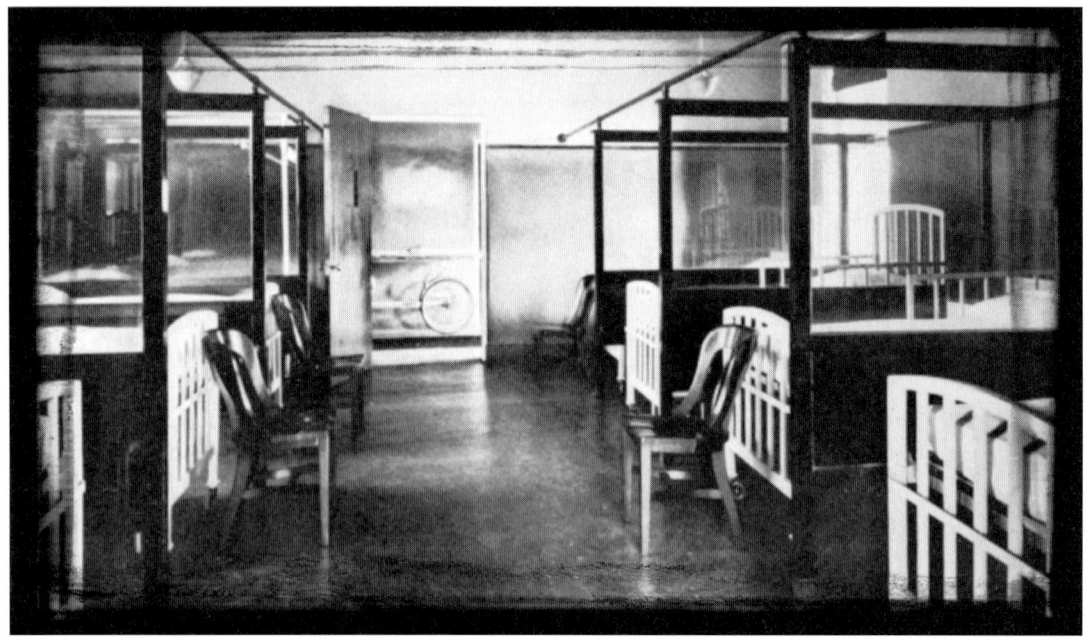

[ACH CHILDREN'S ROOM · 1926]

During the next months the big news was an attempt to build another, competing, hospital on forty-six acres of land south of State Street (in the area between where Parkway Blvd. and Ridgewood Ave. currently exist). The proposal for NovoPathic Hospital consisted of an attempt to sell $2,500,000 in stock in the company in order to build a 400-bed hospital for the treatment of diseases "both general and specific." The hospital was marketing itself as being especially for "men of business" and as such would have "offices" in each room so the men could keep in touch with their business while they were in the hospital.[40]

By June of 1922 news of Alliance City Hospital was good—bids were being accepted for the equipping of the new addition.[41] According to the *Review*, "When completed for use, the City hospital will have a capacity of 100 beds. This will put it on equal rank with any hospital in a city of like size anywhere in Ohio."[42] The hospital was also trying to get a new heating plant built as part of the additions, one that was "of the very latest type."

We don't hear much about the hospital again until 1923. (Interestingly enough, the aforementioned new addition is still not completed.) According to a city audit done in July of 1923, the city had a lot invested in the hospital: more than $300,000 dollars. According to the *Review*, the financial implications of city ownership of the hospital had developed according to the following timeline:

> *On September 14, 1914, the Hospital association, a private organization turned over the property of the association to the city, representing an investment of approximately $20,000. Two years later this valuation was augmented by donations amounting to $5,000. Reeves Brothers' company contributed $1,000, Transue and Williams $1,000, the Buckeye Twist Drill $500, the Morgan Engineering company $1,000, Alliance Machine company $1,000 and the American Steel Foundries $500. … There is outstanding at the present time $290,000 in hospital bonds.*

By October of 1923, the hospital was once again accepting bids for equipping the new addition. The *Review* states that eight concerns were bidding for the right to equip the rooms of the hospital and that the administration would expend the remainder of the $42,000 bond to purchase the equipment. Bidders on the project included the Kauffman-Lattimer Company of Columbus, the Scientific Materials Company of Pittsburgh, and the Pettis, T.W. Cope and Household Supply Company of Alliance.[43]

There was good news from the hospital in October of 1923 – according to minutes of the city council meeting, the hospital was slowly getting back on its feet financially. This was due, the council thought, to the improvements made in the administration of the hospital.

Finally, in November 1923, the new equipment was purchased for the hospital. Bids were spread out to many of the companies. According to a report in the *Alliance Review*, along with the news of the bids came the exciting news that the Alliance Rotary Club was going to build a modern orthopedic ward and provide funding for an orthopedic doctor to help Alliance's crippled children. The ward was to include a "sun parlor, outdoor corridor for fresh air patients and beds for a score or more patients."[44]

By the beginning of 1924, the hospital was starting to see some effects from the tightening of its policy towards charity cases. In the annual business report to city council, prepared and given by Superintendent Fred Walker, the hospital had made a reduction of more than $5,000 in the deficit from hospital operations as compared with the previous year.

Walker also reported the following:

· 845 persons underwent operations.

· 1,266 patients were admitted to the hospital.

· Receipts from these patients came to $57,769.22.

· There were fifty-five deaths at the hospital in the year 1923-24; these included deaths in the emergency room before patients could be admitted to the hospital proper.

· There were 101 births.

· The payroll (excluding medical doctors) for the hospital was roughly $27,000.[45]

In February of 1924, the Rotary Club's bid to finance an orthopedic wing for children was accepted by city council.[46]

In March of 1925 the hospital and the city wrangled over who would pay for necessary repairs. The hospital needed a new hot water tank as well as painting and minor repairs to the nurses' home. The city wanted to float a bond issue for the repairs, but the city auditor, Mr. C.O. Silver, declared that bonds couldn't be used for this purpose and wouldn't authorize the issuance of said bonds.[47] A week later it was reported that the city was required to pay for repairs out of its own hospital funds. The mayor refused, citing the need to use the money to buy supplies for the care of patients, not for repairs.[48] The issue was resolved the following week when the repairs were ordered to come out of the hospital's revenues; the mayor promised, however, to help the hospital make up for any loss the repairs might cause. The council then passed an ordinance to float a bond issue for around half of their original request. This met with Auditor Silver's approval.[49] In other financial news from 1925, the city attempted to force charity cases to pay for their own tests, citing the rising costs of performing the tests, and the overcharging by the laboratory.[50]

The big news in 1925, however, was not related to the hospital's financial situation, nor was it related to the oft-delayed addition.

The strange case of Dr. Albert Wild took over the headlines of the *Alliance Review* for most of the second half of 1925, providing a glimpse into the inner workings of the hospital.

In April of 1925, Dr. Wild went to court to

force the hospital to allow him to "enter." According to the *Review*, Dr. Wild had been barred from the hospital by Charles Smith, Alliance safety director and official head of the hospital. Dr. Wild, court documents claim, was forced to operate with another member of the hospital staff present and was not given his choice of assistants. His suit claims that he wanted simply to be treated like other members of the hospital's professional staff.

The court initially granted Dr. Wild an injunction allowing him access to his patients

[ACH Kids' Playroom · 1926]

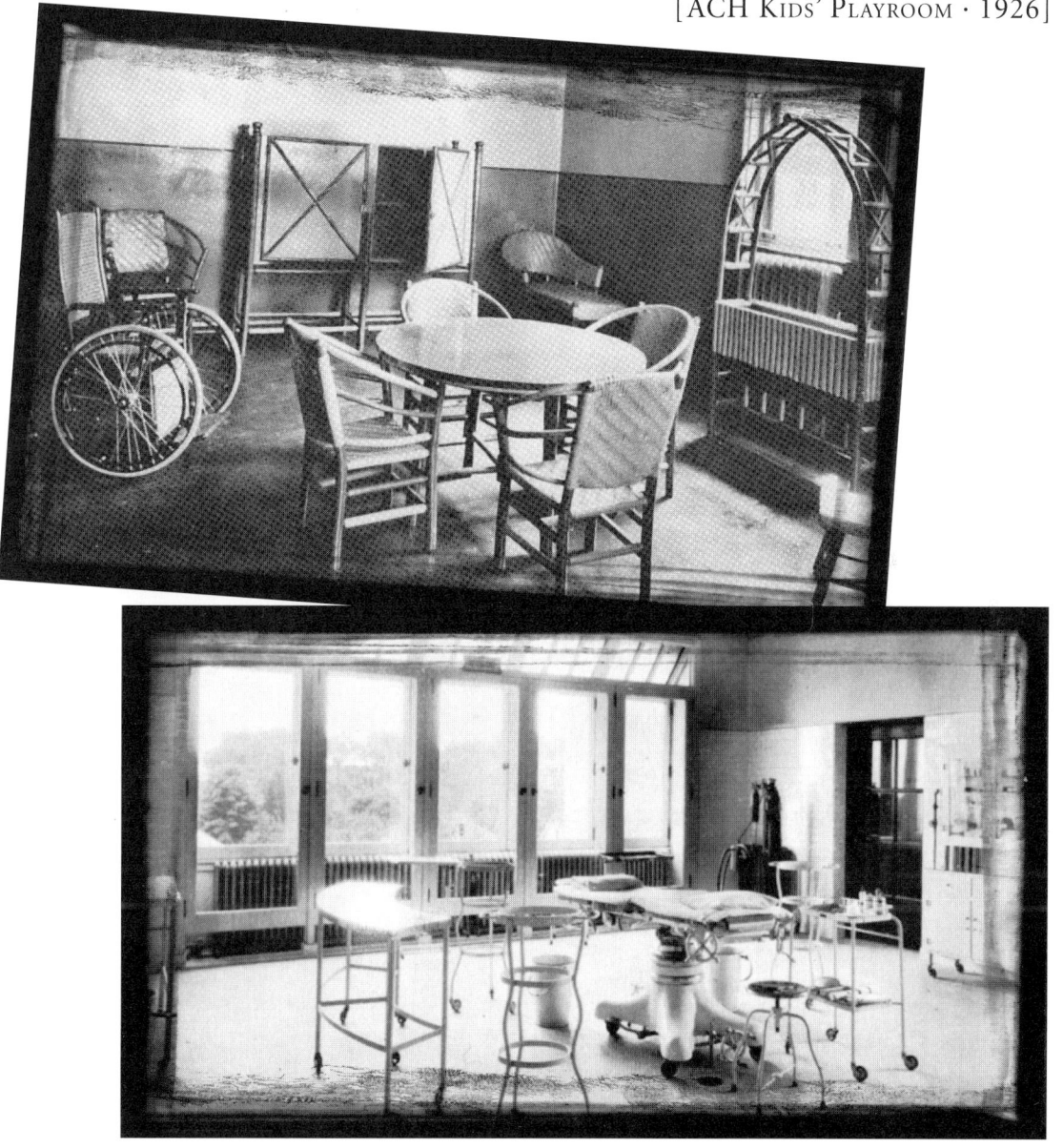

[ACH Operating Room · 1926]

and to the medical and surgical facilities of Alliance City Hospital. The hospital responded by claiming that Dr. Wild had attempted to "take things into his own hands."[51]

Dr. Wild's case then headed to court. Initially the hospital didn't take the case all that seriously. Soon enough the hospital's administration was cited for contempt of court for not providing Dr. Wild and his attorneys with an official set of rules of the hospital. One was eventually provided for him.[52]

The case finally made it to court, much to the delight of the local media. The case became important beyond the boundaries of Dr. Wild and the City Hospital because it was going to set precedent on the right of doctors to use public facilities. Dr. Wild's accusations were that the management of the hospital (the city safety director, the mayor, and the hospital superintendent) was exclusionary and that they had attempted to fire him without the benefit of a hearing. The hospital responded with accusations that Dr. Wild was not a good surgeon. To confirm this, they "produced nurses on the hospital staff who told [of] incidents in which Dr. Wild attempted intimacies with them in the sheltered corridors and rooms of the hospital."[53] Several staff members of the hospital testified as to Dr. Wild's poor surgical technique, although an equal number testified to his ethical and surgical "perfection."

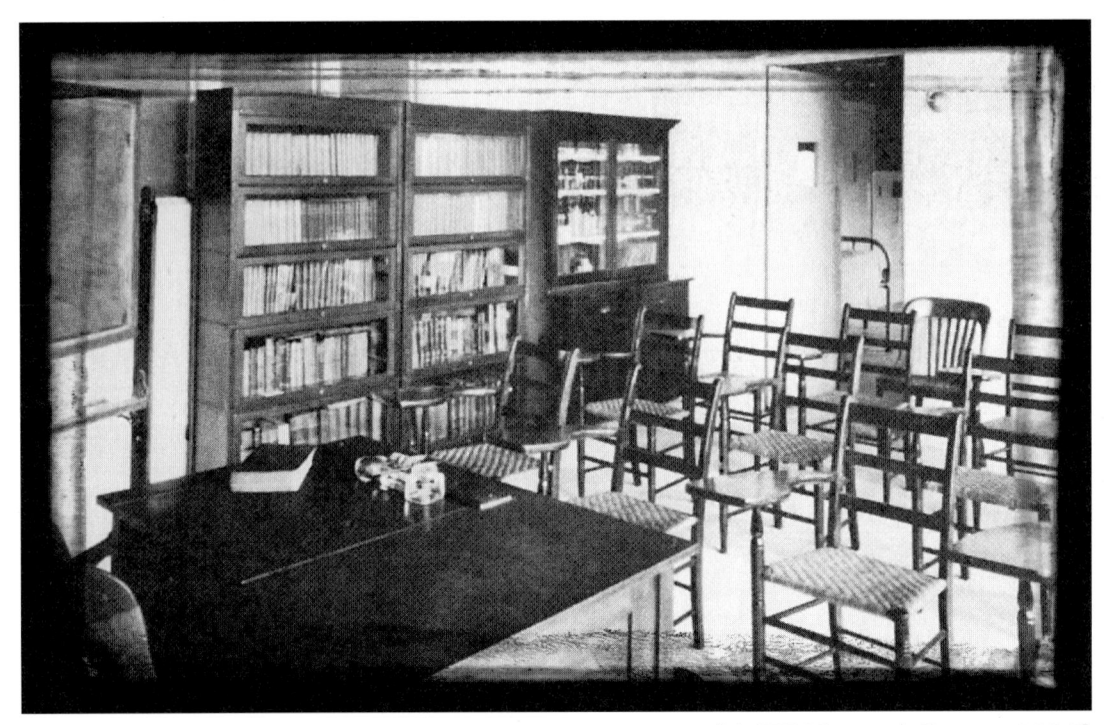

[ACH NURSES' CLASS · 1926]

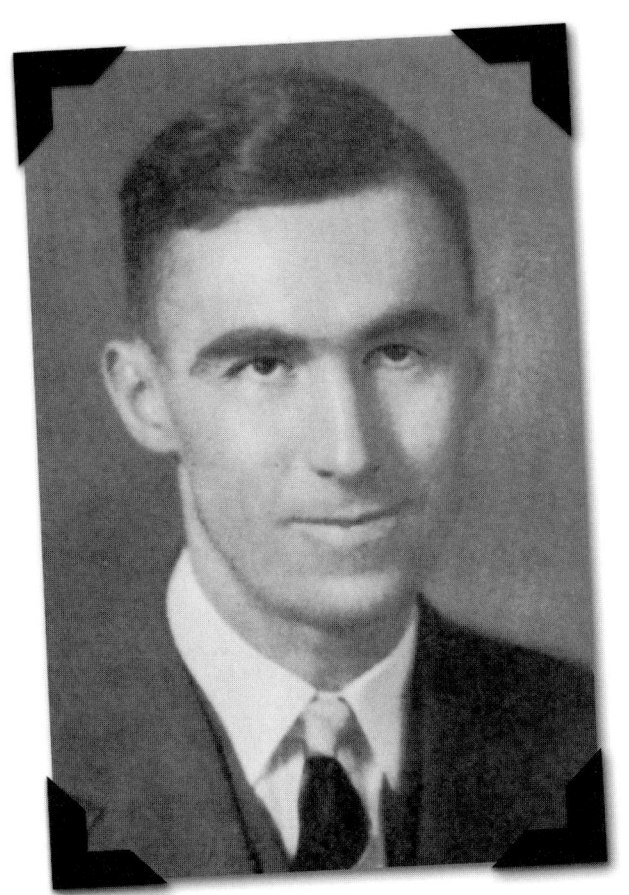

[FRANK W. HOOVER,
SUPERINTENDENT OF HOSPITAL · 1926]

The trial went on for several days, making headlines each day. The major grievance became the clash between Dr. Wild and Superintendent Walker, who, it was reported, allegedly had a screaming match with Dr. Wild while he was performing surgery on a woman for the removal of an abdominal cyst. The case, by this point, had drawn the attention of the Ohio Department of Health. One of their members, a Dr. J.A. Wels, came all the way from Columbus to hear the case "threshed out."[54]

By May of 1925, the case was in the hands of Judge A.W. Agler. Dr. Wild had ended the trial phase of the case by presenting the court with the lengthy brief accusing the hospital of a myriad of abuses including the "unjust and tyrannical" leadership of the superintendent and city safety director.[55] On May 12, the court ruled that Wild's suspension was legal and that he was no longer allowed to practice medicine at Alliance City Hospital. Furthermore, the court upheld the city's position that the

safety director of the city of Alliance has the power to make reasonable rules and regulations for the government of the hospital and the admission of patients thereto; and in making of such rules he may use his discretion as well as in the appointment of the hospital staff for the hospital.[56]

The fight, however, was not over. Soon after Judge Agler's decision was handed down, Wild vowed to appeal "all the way to the supreme court." According to the May 13 *Alliance Review*, Dr. Wild was going to appeal on constitutional grounds, declaring that "I don't intend to let [Agler's] decision stand."[57]

In a strange turn of events, the hospital, after the announcement of the initial decision, offered Wild his privileges back in return for a promise to "abide by the rules of the hospital." In a letter to Wild, Safety Director C.W. Smith wrote:

The Common Pleas Court having sustained the right of the Safety Director of the City of Alliance, Ohio to make and

A CENTURY OF CARING   1920—1930 · 37

enforce the rules for the management of the hospital, your suspension from the use of the hospital heretofore made is limited to thirty days, which will expire June fourth, 1925 (the injunctional order having been in force from April sixteenth to this date). Provided, however, you will give me express assurances that you will in the future conform to the agreement and government of the hospital.[58]

Dr. Wild chose not to take the offer, writing to Safety Director Smith that "whenever you adopt rules that will permit me to practice my profession without self abasement I will gladly comply with them and avail myself of the hospital privileges."[59]

Like many other aspects of history, the story of Dr. Wild fades into obscurity after this last shot across the bow of the hospital. By all accounts, Dr. Wild settled into a comfortable private practice run out of his home on Rockhill Ave.

The last bit of news for 1925 was the naming of Frank Hoover to the superintendency of the hospital. Hoover was a veteran of World War I and, until his hiring by the hospital, an employee of City Savings Bank and Trust Company.

Judging by the headlines in the *Alliance Review*, 1927 was one of the most exciting years in American history. Almost daily, some pilot was attempting to cross some large body of water in an airplane, and in May of 1927, Charles Lindbergh did so, flying from New York to Paris without stopping. This excitement meant a lot of things to the city of Alliance. Soon after Lindbergh's crossing of the Atlantic, Alliance was investigating the need for an airport, and planning for the construction of the Alliance Airplane Company, with the first airplane due to roll off the assembly line in 1929.[60]

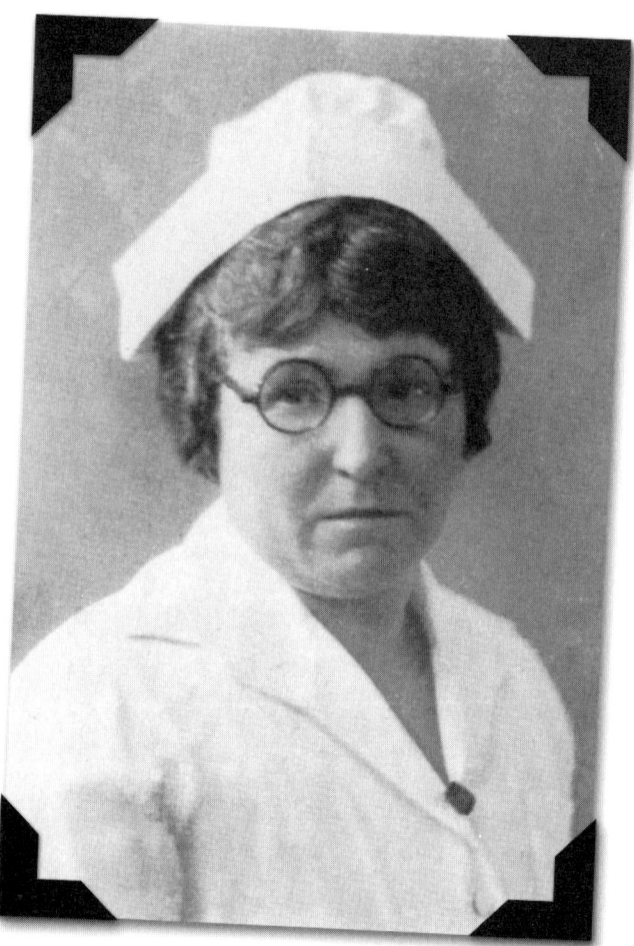

[MISS MARGARET E. TWEEDY, R.N., SUPERINTENDENT OF NURSES · 1926]

These events in 1927 soon became an issue for the hospital. There was, by mid '27, a growing need for an additional hospital annex, including a separate facility for the treatment of contagious diseases and a venereal clinic.[61] These additions, however, were contingent on ever dwindling city funds (much of which were tied up in the airport). Another consequence the lack of funds had for the hospital was the fact that they could not focus on development. For instance, the hospital could not take advantage of an offer from the Kiwanis, who had purchased land on Rice Street for the annex; the hospital was financially unable to build anything on the land and had to back out of the deal.[62] Two days later the *Review* reported that "City Hospital Closes Year with Deficit." The hospital had found the costs of patient upkeep mounting – the cost per patient per day had risen, by 1927, to $4.47; the deficit, by this time, was $4,728.[63] At this time the city was also running at a deficit, and the two deficits combined caused the city to cut the hospital's 1927 budget "to the bone." There would, for instance, only be money to purchase food supplies for the first seven months of the year.[64]

There were, in 1927, also many good things happening to the hospital. The highlight of any year was the graduation of the class of nurses. On May 27, 1927, the nursing school graduated its largest class to date. The commencement address was given by Dr. W.W. Dieterich who stressed the humanitarian mission of the hospital and the nurses' mission to minister to the sick.[65] Ongoing maintenance of the hospital, including the replacing of stair rails, plumbing for the nurses' home and lamps for the rooms, was also a concern.[66]

In August, however, the dire predictions from January came true when the hospital ran out of money to buy food. Since "the City budget [was] tight at the moment," the council voted an extra $5,000 to provide food for the hospital through December.[67] Ironically, while there wasn't enough money to buy food, the first six months of 1927 were the best in the hospital's history; no private room had been vacant for more than two days and revenue was up more than $5,000 from the same time in 1926.[68]

The nursing school and staff were also thriving. There were over 40 nurses on the staff or in training at the nursing school—the most in the history of the hospital. The *Review* gives all of the credit to Miss Margaret Tweedy, superintendent of nurses, for her excellent work in training and recruiting the nurses and forging a "splendid spirit of cooperation with Mt. Union College."[69]

Other good news from the eventful year 1927 included Alliance City Hospital's approval by the American College of Surgeons – something only four hospitals in Stark County could claim (Mercy, Aultman, and Massillon City were the others).[70] In late October, the

Review reported that the maternity ward was repainted and replastered with money left in trust by Mr. Simon Hartzell.

In the year-end report for 1927, more good news: the death rate for the hospital was down 1.6%. The deficit was down to $3,506.11.[71] The new superintendent, Dr. Hoover, was calling 1927 the best year in the hospital's history. Things were looking up.

The years 1928-1929 were relatively normal for the hospital—the nursing school continued to receive high marks from outside observers, including "warm praise" from the State Inspector of Schools of Nursing for Superintendent Margaret Tweedy and the work she was doing.[72] For most of the rest of the decade, the nursing school was filled to capacity and even had to turn applications down.

The hospital continued to purchase equipment and modernize as well. In April 1928 the hospital considered buying radios for every room, the claim being that "air programs are found beneficial to patients." There is no indication as to whether the Hospital bought the radios or not.[73] In October 1928, the hospital made its most important equipment purchase yet when it bought new X-ray machines from the Victor X-ray Company of Chicago. The contract called for the installation of "two complete units of most modern design at a cost of between $8,800 and $9,000." The machines to be installed consisted of "one horizontal Buckey table for fluoroscopic and radiographic work and one tilt table."[74]

The hospital continued to get high marks from the State College of Surgeons, gaining approval in both 1928 and 1929. The article "Alliance City Hospital on 'Preferred List'" in the October 12 edition of the *Review* sheds some interesting light on medicine in the late twenties. According to the State College of Surgeons,

> *Eleven years ago the patient remained in the hospital twenty to twenty-four days, on the average, whereas today he remains only twelve to fourteen days in the same hospital in the same condition. Eleven years ago seventy to ninety persons per thousand treated in hospital died, whereas today this has been reduced to twenty to thirty on the average in standardized hospitals. Eleven years ago eighteen persons out of every hundred undergoing major operations died, but today this has dropped to three or less, due to more competent surgery and the development of new methods of anesthesia and improved technique and procedures.*

In his annual report to city council at the end of 1928, Superintendent Hoover listed the hospital as treating 1,317 patients at an average cost of $5.23 per patient per day (an average stay of 10.7 days was also reported). There were 113 births and 95 deaths. Hoover cited a water softener and physiotherapy equipment as projected needs for 1929.[75]

With the growing domestic financial crises—including the stock market crash of October 1929; the "hoarding" crisis; and the closing of several local and national banks, news about the hospital in late 1929 and early 1930 is scarce. There is no information, as there usually was, about nursing school graduations or the hospital's annual report. In fact, the only real information about the hospital to be found for mid to late 1929 comes in through sort of a side entrance: in May 1929, the X-ray storage rooms at two of the country's major hospitals, the Cleveland Clinic and San Francisco General blew up; the explosion at the Cleveland Clinic killed over 100 people, at least one of whom was an Alliance native. Alliance City Hospital was immediately pronounced safe from this kind of potential disaster, with Safety Director Norman Fetters and Chief of Staff Frank Hoover claiming that "all X-ray storage facilities are now of the most current construction."[76]

The final bit of news about the hospital at the end of this most turbulent decade was the good news that it had maintained its good standing in the annual College of Surgeons review. Of the 200 hospitals in Ohio at the time, only 86 were on said list. Local hospitals not on the list included Portage County Hospital in Ravenna and East Liverpool City Hospital.[77]

The hospital ended one of the oddest decades on record much as it began—in a moderate amount of debt but doing exceptional work and continuing to serve, and make proud, the citizens of Alliance.

A CENTURY OF CARING

1930-1940

1930—1940

It is difficult, I imagine, for someone who did not live through the American Economic Depression of 1929-40 to understand the way in which it touched nearly every aspect of every life in America — in both big cities and small towns. The incredible optimism with which Herbert Hoover had been elected in November 1928 was dashed almost immediately upon his taking office in 1929. The disbelief with which federal, state, and local governments treated the ever-expanding economic crisis took an already bad problem (there had been several successive years of drought in the mid and far west and an expanding economic crisis in Europe due in part to unpaid reparations from World War I) and made it even worse.[78]

Alliance City Hospital serves as an excellent microcosm of the effect of the Depression on a small town in America. The hospital headed into the thirties optimistic despite increasing evidence that Alliance was in the middle of an economic disaster[79]; it ended the decade with a smaller nursing school and slashed budgets across the board. But it managed to survive a decade that saw many Alliance businesses fail. As we will see, this is a testament to the high regard in which the hospital was then held by the city; for when the chips were down, the city would always, without exception (although not without a little argument) do the right thing.

By early 1930 the unemployment rate in Alliance was roughly 30%, almost 5% higher than the country as a whole. Despite this staggering unemployment rate, the hospital continued to operate as it had during the economic boom of the mid-twenties. The first time the hospital is mentioned by the Alliance *Review* in 1930 is the proud announcement

A CENTURY OF CARING

that the hospital was going to host the annual District One meeting of the Ohio State Nurses' Association.[80] This was followed by the excellent news that Superintendent Frank Hoover had been named president of the Ohio Hospital Association.[81] The hospital was also, during this time, looking for more room for the nurses and worrying about how to best celebrate National Hospital Day.

Perhaps one sign of the impending financial difficulties to come was the ill-fated National Hospital Day book drive of 1930. According to the *Review*, there was a great need for a library branch at the hospital. The hospital solicited donations of books and money (they needed around $100 to cover some of the start-up costs) during the week immediately after National Hospital Day. The drive was overseen by the Y.M.C.A.'s Ward Gray as well as members of the City's Pioneer Club.[82]

The drive was not successful. In fact, it was the first unsuccessful drive of any sort in the hospital's thirty-year history. According to H.B. Sohn, head of the Carnegie Free Library (now Rodman Public Library), less than $40 and fewer than 500 books had been donated (they had been hoping for $100 and a minimum of 1000 books). The hospital was undaunted, but the failure of the book drive was a harbinger of things to come.[83]

Despite the economic situation, the hospital continued to be a center for excellence and innovation — in August of 1930, for instance, the hospital adopted the footprint system for identifying babies in order to "prevent an Alliance repetition of the Bamberger-Watkins case in Chicago."[84]

Perhaps the most important event of 1930 was the resignation of longtime hospital superintendent, Frank Hoover. Hoover resigned in August 1930, in order to take the superintendent's position at a pair of hospitals in Elyria for "a substantial increase in salary." Hoover's very productive tenure at the hospital had seen the installation of a modern X-ray machine, expansion of the school for nurses, and the establishment of the "crippled children's facility" sponsored by the Rotary.[85]

Hoover's story is an interesting one, particular, it would seem, to his time. The *Alliance Review* reports that he had moved to Alliance in 1905 to be "chore boy for R.M. Scranton … [caring] for the horses and [performing] duties about the Scranton home to work his way through high school." He later attended Alliance High School, graduating with the class of 1908. He attended Mount Union College and served in the air corps during World War I and returned home to become circulation manager of a Zanesville newspaper. He eventually returned to Alliance and became a teller at City Savings Bank. He was then tapped to be superintendent of the hospital and eventually became president of the Ohio Hospital Association.

Hoover was replaced by Alfred H. Simmons of New York City, who came to Alliance in late September.[86] Simmons immediately instituted some positive changes for the hospital, including weekly meetings with the health commission and the mayor and a fund drive to have "5000 people to offer one dollar apiece" in a campaign to raise $5000 for the hospital. In his appeal, Simmons wrote:

> *Ask yourself the question: "What have I ever done for our hospital?" Will your answer to this question be one that satisfies or will you find you could have done your bit for the most important institution of the community, a place where life and death are being fought, where care, attention, steadiness, and humanity are constantly demanded.*[87]

The fund drive got off to a roaring success with the donation of $500 by local businessman, W.E. Davis, "in appreciation of the services the hospital had afforded him while a patient there."[88] Interestingly enough, there is very little information about how the fund drive turned out; the hospital soon turned its attention to building a new facility for the nurses and then, later in October, the first of many disastrous budget problems that were to plague the hospital throughout the thirties.

The nurses' home had, in November 1930, received a terrible review by the state building inspector and was in desperate need of both repair (to the existing facility) and expansion (to a larger facility).[89] Superintendent Simmons went before the city council in December 1930, in an effort to persuade them to buy the land directly behind the hospital (at the time the land was owned by the Kiwanis Club). Simmons also went before the Kiwanis in an effort to get the land donated.[90]

Before the expansion of the nurses' home could be completed, however, more mundane matters intruded: a city audit of the hospital's books found the hospital short by nearly $9,750. Superintendent Simmons claimed in a meeting with city council that this was normal procedure for hospitals (to run a deficit at the end of the year) because of the thin margin of profit a hospital can stand to make.[91] Two days later, however, the *Alliance Review* was reporting that city council was not going to give the hospital the money it needed to continue operation on into 1931 and that they were not going to be able to purchase the additional land needed for the nurses' home. Eventually city council provided $7,459 in operating funds for the remainder of 1930, although they put the superintendent "on the grill" for a larger portion of the meeting and warned him that he "must live within his income in 1931."[92]

Whether it was the stress of fighting with city hall, or the disappointment of not being able to fix the nurses' residence, or something more personal, A.H. Simmons, the superintendent of the hospital for little more than six months, greeted the city council in January of 1931 by resigning his post and moving to Florida.[93]

Needless to say, the city and the hospital staff were surprised by this sudden and unexpected turn of events and pledged to work together to see their way through the emergency situation. It is unclear to this day if there is a relationship between Simmons leaving his post and the mysterious $8,998.56 overdraft found in the accounts for 1930 that forced the city to finish its year in the red for the first time in memory. The dire straits that the hospital was in mirrored the city's economic problems: according to the *Review*, the city's tax receipts were down by more than $10,000 over 1929, while the hospital's receipts were down nearly $3,000.[94]

While all of this was going on, the hospital managed to hire a new superintendent: Mr. Harold W. Wagner of 1435 Robinwood Road, former co-owner of Graham and Wagner Monuments. Mr. Wagner was a local man, born and raised in New Philadelphia and educated at Western Reserve University. He had been a resident of Alliance for the eight years before being named hospital superintendent.[95]

Mr. Wagner took over a hospital that was in "splendid shape," according to members of city council. Mr. Wagner immediately moved to mend fences with city council. At his first report to city council, Wagner gave a detailed analysis of why he thought the hospital was losing money. According to Wagner, 7% of the hospital cases were flat-out charity cases, and another 2% were cases where the patient had promised to pay but for some reason would not; as well, there were several car accident cases in which the victim couldn't or wouldn't pay. This was the cause, Wagner argued, for an almost $1,500 deficit per month between collections and expenditures.[96]

That same year Wagner also saw the hospital remain accredited by the Council of Medical Education and Hospitals of the American Medical Association. The nursing school was also cited as a reason for excellence.[97]

1931's "Hospital Day" drew over 300 visitors (a record) to the hospital to hear speeches and witness presentations by hospital staff. The visitors were heard to "manifest genuine enthusiasm over the tidy appearance of the hospital and remarked at the manner in which the institution is being run."[98] Later that same month another record class of nurses graduated from the nursing school, hearing an address by the Reverend H.K. Hillberry on the subject of "calling and character," and a speech by Dr. L.T. Headland of Mount Union College.[99]

The increasing financial squeeze of the early thirties found the hospital forced to get increasingly creative and vigilant about its collection of unpaid bills. Several times during the early thirties, the city solicitor of Alliance would be ordered by city council to "get tough" with those who would not/could not pay their bills.[100] And while this worked in a limited manner, it did not go nearly far enough to reduce the more than $10,000 deficit that the hospital was running by May 1931. Later that same year the hospital decided not to treat or admit citizens of Brown Township/Carroll County until their local governments had cleared up their bills amounting to $85.50.[101]

Another attempt to remedy the poor financial situation was to ask the state to reimburse the hospital for "indigent automobile cases." According to a report made by Superintendent Wagner to the State Hospital Association, these car crashes were costing hospitals an average of $1,500 per year. What Wagner envisioned, he reports, was something akin to workman's compensation where the hospital would care for the injured motorist without worrying about payment.[102]

Money issues consumed the remainder of 1931. In September the city went to the voters with a levy to raise money to continue to operate the hospital and in the same month the nursing school reduced its staff by two and its freshman class admissions by three.[103]

In October, Stark County passed a resolution that it would aid the four main hospitals in the area — Aultman, Mercy, Massillon, and Alliance City, with money raised from county bonds. According to the November 13 Alliance Review, the hospital stood to receive a total of $6,000 from the county. While this helped erase some of the old debt from the books, the increasing depression was, according to Superintendent Wagner, making collections of present bills more difficult.

By the end of 1931 Mr. Wagner had the hospital under control. In his final report of the year, Wagner told the city council that the hospital was going to come in $500 under budget due mainly to the new rule that patients had to make satisfactory financial arrangements before treatment would be considered.[104]

1932 saw no improvement in the somewhat chaotic financial situation of the hospital (indeed, it simply mirrors the situation of the city, the state, and the country as a whole). In mid-February, four nurses (Ruth Binder, Goldie West, Ella Costello, and Mary Wright) quit and several others went on "staggered" schedules in an effort to keep the hospital adequately staffed while at the same time lowering the annual operating costs. Cooks and housekeepers were also asked to stagger their work schedules.[105]

Superintendent Wagner made several other suggestions at this time, including the recommendation that the nursing school be closed, that student nurses be let go, and that graduate nursing students be brought in to replace regular nurses. According to the Review,

With these facts at their fingertips and with taxpayers clamoring for a reduction in expenses at every point possible, the superintendent, mayor, director, and finance committee of council have worked out the economy program.

Within days, however, and due in no small part to the vocal objection of the citizens, the nurses were brought back and all discussion of eliminating the nursing school was declared "premature." Wagner, however, in hiring the nurses back, took the opportunity to revise the administration of the hospital, creating the position of business manager for himself (in addition to his job as superintendent) and directress of nurses.[106]

By 1932 the watchword all throughout Alliance was "pay slash." City council members were "donating" two weeks of their pay every six months, Mount Union College professors had accepted a 40% pay cut, city employees had seen their salaries cut by 10%, police and fire departments started a policy of taking "payless vacations", and the hospital nursing staff was reduced from thirty-three to twenty.[107] At this same time, however, the hospital was able to reduce its general operating fund by almost $6,000, much of which was due to the excellent management by Superintendent/Business Manager Wagner.[108]

In mid-1932, the daily patient count averaged forty-one and the average cost-per-day was $5.20. Both of these figures were down slightly (9%) from the year before. Both Wagner and city council attributed the decrease in costs to Wagner's "rigid economies".[109]

By August the city and the hospital were continuing their economic decline. On the same day the *Alliance Review* reported that city employees were being asked to take an additional 10% pay cut (their second in six months), it reported that the three ranking members of the nursing school's administration quit. No reasons were given for the resignations and no effort was made to replace the nurses.[110] A week later one replacement was hired when Mrs. Mary Taylor left her position as secretary of the Alliance Woman's Club and took over the position of superintendent of nurses.[111]

By the end of 1932 the nursing school was again in danger. According to reports, an ordinance was introduced at the last meeting of city council of 1932 to discontinue the nursing school in order to save the city $10,650.14 (at the time the city was over $107,000 in debt, due mainly to ever-decreasing tax receipts).[112]

In response to the continual tinkering by city council, Superintendent Wagner asked, in late December, that the hospital be removed from city control in order to "divorce the City hospital from political influence."[113] According to the proposal, a hospital commission would be created to supervise the institution. The commission would be made up of three staff members, three council members, and three citizens (chosen by the other six). The commission would "control the hospital, supervising expenditures and performing other similar functions."

The hospital was the sole discussion point of the first council meeting of 1933. The reappointment of Mr. Wagner as superintendent,[114] the discussion of the proposed governance structure, and the fate of the nursing school were all discussed at great length. According to the *Review*, "Figures were quoted, petitions introduced, resolutions adopted and an old-fashioned town meeting discussion developed Tuesday night as city council gave consideration to problems arising at the City hospital."[115]

In another move, two days later, city solicitor, Harry Wykoff, declared that the changes in governance proposed by the hospital were not legal and that, according to state code, "the entire management of the city hospital is vested in the safety-service director, subject to the ordinances of council."[116]

At the second city council meeting of 1933, no action was taken on the realignment of the hospital governance, but, in a surprise move, the council unanimously voted down the measure to discontinue the nursing school. The move to keep the training school was led by Councilman J.R. Hoiles who stated at the meeting that "we [council and the hospital] have worked out plans by which we can make a saving almost as great as by suspending the school, and we think it better to continue the school."[117]

1934 saw the city busy registering the unemployed for relief; the WPA providing government building jobs (Alliance saw many roads paved through this program); and Hugh "Ironpants" Johnson and the NRA deciding which businesses got to fly the "blue eagle." After the struggles in 1933 over hospital governance and the nursing school, it was undoubtedly a relief to many that 1934 was a year without a major event for the hospital, and except for the now yearly announcements about the nursing school graduation, National Hospital Day, and the reaccreditation of the hospital by the Ohio Hospital Association, Alliance City Hospital managed to stay out of the newspaper entirely except for the relatively minor announcement of the creation of a new executive position of business manager (a position created informally by Superintendent Wagner and held in tandem with the position of superintendent). According to a story in the Alliance *Review*, the business manager would be involved in looking after "expenditures, collections, purchases, and the care of materials." According to Mayor Guy Abbot, this position was created "to make the hospital as good financially as professionally."[118] The salary was set at $125 a month and was approved unanimously by city council.

A month later, Mr. C.E. Sperow, of Ridgewood Ave., was named business manager. Mr. Sperow had been active in the management of the Suburban Power Company and before that was in management with the Westinghouse Electric Company.[119]

In January 1935, the city began studying plans for relief of the hospital, calling it a "financially insolvent institution".[120] A committee of doctors was formed to study the "extremely serious financial conditions facing the city and hospital."[121] Following closely on the heels of this committee report was the resignation of C.E. Sperow as finance director and the appointment of William Harrington to replace him. Harrington came to the hospital after serving as an accountant at City Savings and Trust Company and as adjutant of the local American Legion post.[122]

For most of 1935 discussions continued between the hospital and city council about how to achieve solvency for the hospital; several interesting ideas were tried, none more so than the hiring of the Jones-Williamson Rodeo to put on a charity show at Bluebell field, with all proceeds going to the hospital for the purchasing of supplies and materials.[123] The rodeo was slated to have "20 features out of the West." Items which were to be purchased with the proceeds included

> sheets, pillow cases, woolen blankets, window blinds, mattresses for nursery cribs, nursery supplies, x-ray films, bandages, gauze, transfusion sets, towels, washcloths, and operating room supplies.

According to a spokesperson for the hospital, many of the aforementioned items had not been replaced in years and were literally "tattered and torn."[124] The public was very much behind this fundraising effort, with the city of Sebring taking the lead by buying 950 tickets and challenging the city of Alliance to do the same. Acts slated to appear included Frank Daniels and his horse "Cody" (who were going to leave Alliance and head off to Hollywood for a sixteen-week job with Fox motion pictures); "Tony the Wop" and his mule "Susie"; and Miss Lola Hunt, one of the nation's best equestriennes.[125] The rodeo finally went off; not, however, without a hitch: the first two nights were rained out and the rodeo was booked to do two shows on Sunday to make up for the loss. Eventually the hospital cleared, after expenses, $275 from the benefit.[126]

Even with the infusion of money from the rodeo, the hospital still needed help. In November, Mr. Harrington and Dr. George King, chief of staff of the hospital, made appeals to the Kiwanis Club for money. The Kiwanis members voted to support a levy for the hospital including taking out advertisements in the *Review* and providing speakers to appear in every school in the city to drum up support for it.[127]

A one mill operating levy slated to raise approximately $25,000 failed to pass by less than one percent (a levy at the time needed 65% of the vote, the hospital levy received a clear majority but only 64.5% of the vote).[128] To alleviate the hospital from the debt accrued by the difference between collections and operating expenses, finance director Harrington instituted a policy of interviewing patients before they were treated to ascertain their ability to pay before receiving services.[129]

Another organization was formed in 1935; this one, the Hospital Auxiliary, remains with us today. According to the hospital's records, the auxiliary was founded "Early in the month of October 1935" by Mrs. Fay Asherman, Mrs. Karl Fiegenschuh, Mrs. Harry Roderick, and Mrs. Walter Webb.[130] The first fundraiser held by the auxiliary was "Donation Days" in which a number of items, including canned food, bars of soap, vegetables, coffee, and tea were collected.

The levy became an issue again in 1936, this time passing by a "decisive majority" in the May primary election.[131] Then disaster struck: due to a new state law prohibiting a levy that would last for more than two years from being voted upon in a primary election, the hospital levy was struck down by Ohio Attorney General John Bricker and the first series of tax collections were refunded to citizens.[132] For a variety of reasons, including a better collections-to-operations ratio by the hospital's financial office, the levy was not placed on the November ballot.[133] In a further effort to raise money and reduce debt, the hospital approached the state and asked them to pay for indigent patients through the Cary Relief Act; they also asked the county to help pay salaries and maintenance.[134]

The city was not feeling benevolent at this point. Many on city council were upset at having to constantly bail the hospital out with money from the general fund and the payment of interest on the bonds raised in the twenties to build the addition had become a yearly drain on city finances.[135] The hospital even asked the WPA to help them make repairs and build a new nurses' home and school; and while the building of a new home was rejected by the WPA, $2,500 in repairs were authorized and completed in mid 1937.[136]

Soon after the repairs on the home were completed, the state requested that if the nursing school were to continue in operation, the course of instruction be increased and "sanitary facilities improved."[137] The curriculum requirements (increased training in chemistry and biology) were easily met by Mount Union College; the isolation of the obstetrical ward and repairs to the plumbing required by the state were more difficult — the money for these two items would have to come out of the city's general fund which was, as was everything else in 1937, at an all-time low.

In December 1937 city council voted to pay for the necessary repairs ($1,200) and to pay the tuition of the nurses to Mount Union College ($7.50 per semester hour). These moves met the requirements of the state and once again the nursing school found itself in business for another year.[138]

In 1938 the city made its most drastic cuts

yet: the "discharge of 10 policemen and as many firemen ... immediate closing of the parks and operation of the City Hospital only until November 1."[139] City council voted to ask the residents of the city to help with yet another levy, this time a general city operating levy, to be voted upon that November. Another bond issue was approved for voting in 1939, not without controversy, however, this time about the quality of meals at the hospital.[140]

Despite the financial crisis, the hospital was still doing outstanding work. In April, 1938, the nursing school was given the highest rating by the Ohio State Nurses' Association, who cited the hospital as "one of the pacesetters for the state."[141] The nursing school managed to graduate classes of seven, five, and six respectively during the years 1937, 1938, and 1939.[142]

The hospital, like much in America, barely survived the thirties. It survived, however, a much-changed institution. During the thirties the hospital became a leaner operation, hiring a finance director, suing for collections, creating an interview system to see if patients could pay their bills before they were treated, and working with the state and the county to receive money for the treatment of the indigent, those hurt in automobile accidents, and those unable, for any other reason, to pay their bills. The nursing school, despite its continued high ratings by the state, faced an almost annual threat of closure, yet managed to do excellent work. The next decade would find the hospital well positioned to take advantage of the changes it had made during the thirties to become a booming institution central to the life of the city of Alliance.

A CENTURY OF CARING

1940—Present

1940 – Present[143]

In 1940, Franklin Delano Roosevelt was running for president against Wendell Willkie, a surprise sixth ballot choice at the Republican national convention; America was debating isolationism and Lend-Lease politics and marveling at FDR's last prewar budget, which had topped out at 8.8 billion dollars. Scientists were discovering various uses for plasma while people were traveling by car from Indianapolis to Chicago in six hours. Synthetic hose started to replace silk stockings, and *Gangbusters* and *The Lone Ranger* were the most popular radio shows.[144]

The primary stories of Alliance City Hospital during the first few years of the forties were, as usual, money and staffing. In 1942, for instance, hospital superintendent, John Cheeks, left for the war and was replaced by longtime Mount Union College employee, Robert Carr.[145] Carr had been business manager of Mount Union College for twenty-eight years. His salary was set at $175 per month.

In 1943, the hospital went before the city with a request for $700,000 in bond money to be used in the following ways: $150,000 for repairs to the nurses' home; $100,000 for a new laundry and boiler room; $50,000 for alterations to the existing physical plant of the hospital; $400,000 for a new addition to the hospital.[146] Later that year a discussion of a $2,000,000 combined hospitals and schools levy was discussed. According to Superintendent Carr, the money from the combined levy would be used for an addition to the hospital that would provide seventy-five more beds and a new nurses' home. The bond issue had the support of both city council and the chamber of commerce, but it did not have much popular support and would not pass, despite repeated attempts, until after the war.

In another wartime setback, the hospital, in 1943, was, for the first time, only conditionally reapproved by the American College of Surgeons due to wartime shortages. According to Dr. Irwin Abell, head of the College of Surgeons, "The 1942 survey disclosed that a few hospitals previously approved are not meeting minimum standard today. Consequently approval was withheld or a provisional rating given."[147] The main problem at the hospital, according to Mayor Floyd Senn, was the loss of staff, especially nurses, to the war effort. The report went on to say that

> great shifts of population due to new and relocated war industries and establishment of large military encampments have caused excessive demands for hospital service in some communities and there is increasing danger of lowered standards in the effort to care for more patients than the depleted staffs can properly serve.

Another issue that the hospital needed to deal with during the war years included a consideration of the size and effectiveness of the nurses' home, which, it seems, was constantly under review. According to an article in the May 18, 1942 edition of the *Alliance Review*, "City council Monday night instructed its hospital committee to make a preliminary study of the possibilities for a new or improved nurses' home."[148] City council spent most of 1943 arguing about the nurses' home—especially whether Alliance needed a new nurses' home first, to enable it to attract more nurses, or whether the city needed new nurses in order to justify the building of a larger, newer home.

Towards the end of the war, the Alliance City Hospital, in what turned out to be its most controversial public move to date, attempted to change the way it was governed—to move out from under control of the city and form its own governing board. Previous attempts had been thwarted by city council, the state attorney general, or the hospital board itself. According to the *Alliance Review*, the hospital's move towards a trusteeship form of governance had the backing of many different factions. This move was supported by Dr. G.L. King, the new head of the medical staff at the hospital. Dr. King's concerns, upon election, were the need for a more self-supporting hospital and more hospital beds. In a speech to the Hospital Auxiliary in 1943, Dr. King mentioned that the new "hospital insurance" was causing more people than ever before to use hospitals and thus requiring facilities to be bigger and more self-sufficient.[149] Despite the public shouting and hand-wringing over the governance change, it would be several more years before anything happened.

Around the same time that Dr. King took over the medical staff, Miss Martha Wunschel was named superintendent of nursing and directress of the school of nursing.[150] Miss Wunschel came to Alliance from Zanesville,

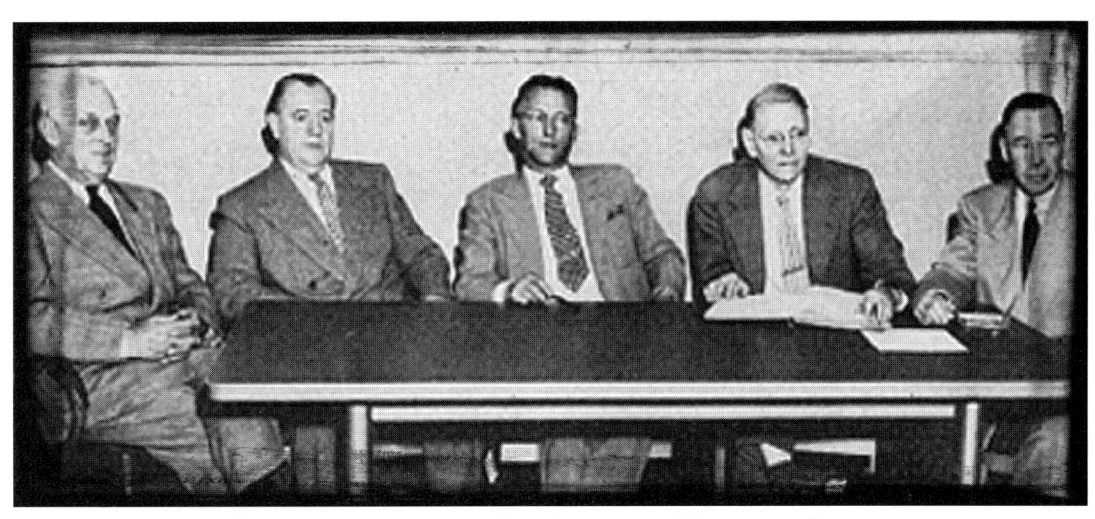

[MEMBERS OF THE ACH BOARD OF HOSPITAL COMMISSIONERS, 1947,
*who directed construction of the new Alliance City Hospital addition are shown above,
left to right: Edgar H. Turkle, Ben A. Tuttle, Mayor Harley R. Ewing, D.M. Armstrong,
and Dr. Harry L. Weaver. The mayor by virtue of his office is Chairman of the Board.*]

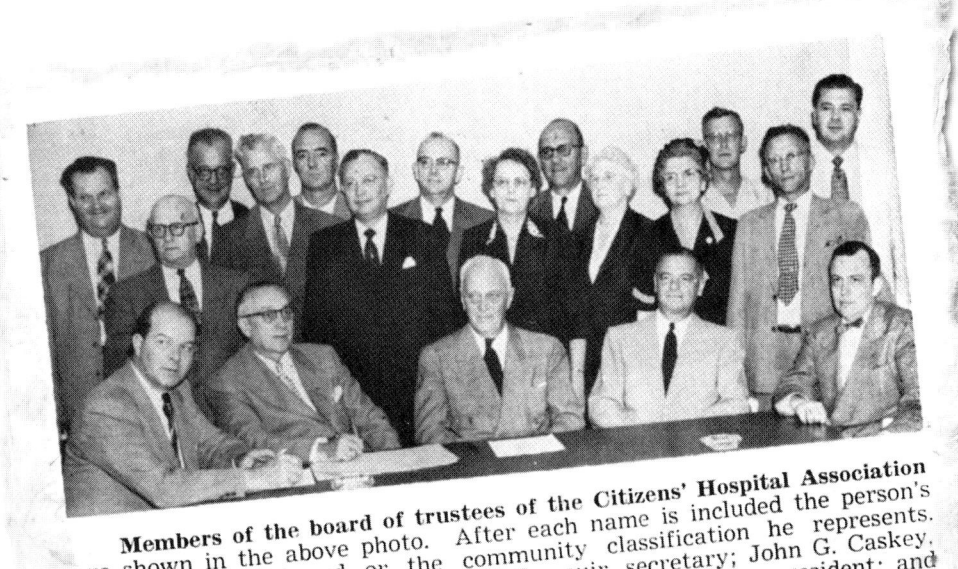

Members of the board of trustees of the Citizens' Hospital Association are shown in the above photo. After each name is included the person's position on the board or the community classification he represents. Seated, left to right, are: Ralph E. Kenmuir, secretary; John G. Caskey, treasurer; Edgar H. Turkle, president; Joseph McFee, vice president; and Robert B. Carey, hospital administrator. Standing, left to right, are: Kimmel Brown, City Council; Harold G. Hubbard, C.I.O.; H. Gordon Robertson, industry; Roy J. Fullmer, business and professional; Willard R. James, at-large; James G. Eardley, Sebring; C. Harold Saffell, Lexington Township; Mrs. R. T. Strauss, at-large; R. J. Van Abel, at-large; Mrs. Karl F. Fiegenschuh, Hospital Auxiliary; Mrs. John Baker, Knox Township; William Anderson, A. F. of L.; Harley R. Ewing, mayor; and John R. Liber, Washington Township. Not present was William H. Morgan, Jr., at-large.

A CENTURY OF CARING   *1940—Present* · 59

OH, where she had been head of nursing at Bethesda Hospital. Before that she had worked in Pontiac, MI, Minneapolis, MN, and hospitals in North Carolina, Texas, and New Jersey. Her undergraduate degree and nursing degree both came from the University of Minnesota. In February 1945, the oft-discussed plan to place the hospital under a trusteeship became, yet again, the talk of the town. According to the *Review*,

> Details of a carefully prepared plan for placing the operations of the City Hospital under a trusteeship in an effort to make the institution tops in efficiency and service in this part of the nation, were unfolded and approved Friday night by the executive committee of the Alliance Betterment Council.[151]

The committee that drew up the plan consisted of F.K. Donaldson, M.E. Rhue, and H.E. Fennerty, with the assistance of hospital expert, Dr. Robin Buerki, of Philadelphia. The plan featured the following items:

· The city would lease the hospital to the

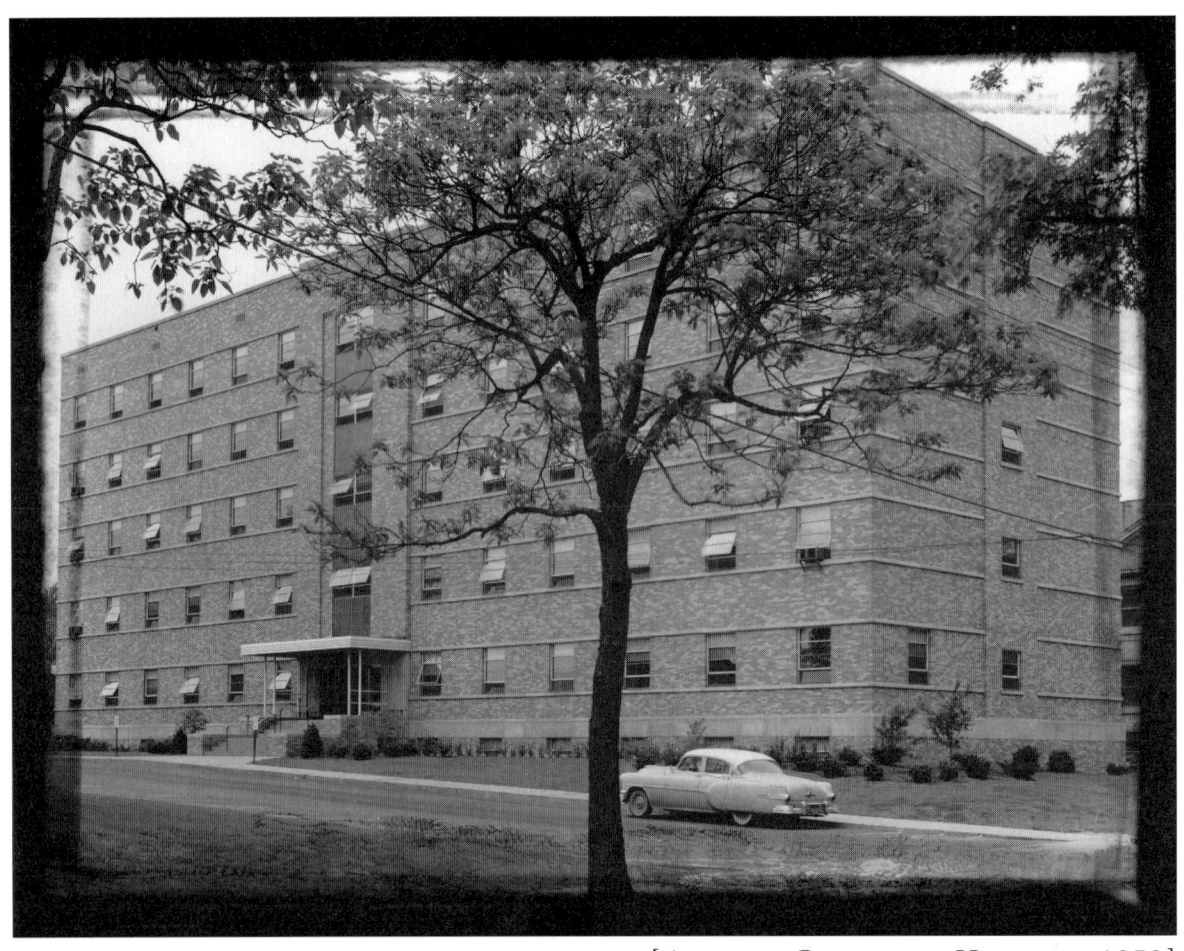

[ALLIANCE COMMUNITY HOSPITAL · 1950]

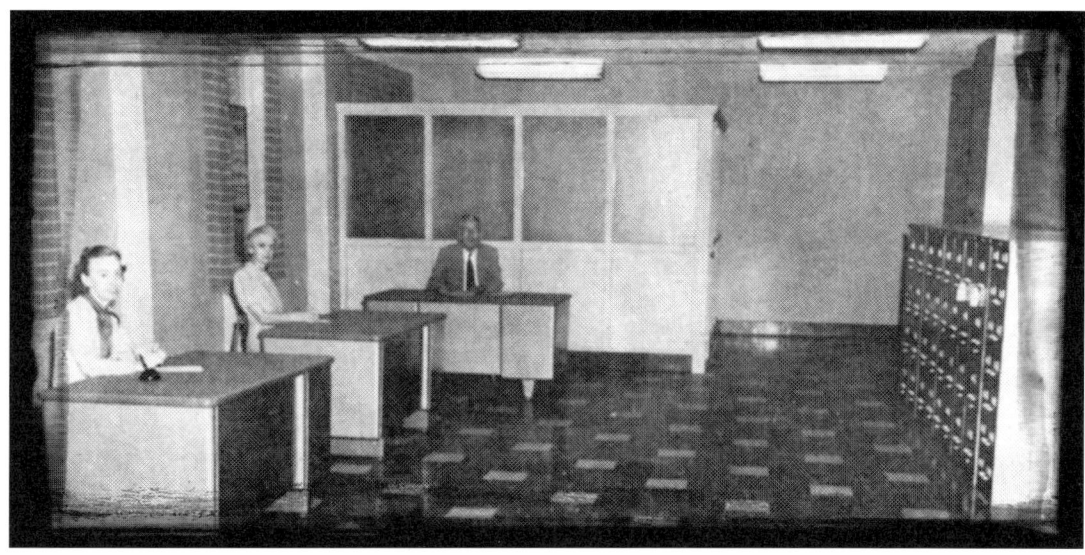

[ACH BUSINESS OFFICE · 1953]

Alliance Hospital Association.

· The association would consist of all persons who acquired a membership by contributing from $5 to $100 a year to the hospital (with all funds from this source being used for capital improvements).

· The association would have complete control of the hospital, electing a trustees' board which in turn would choose a competent and experienced administrator to direct the institution.

· There would be a trustees' board of 15 members elected from the membership and one member named by city council. The medical staff of the hospital would not be eligible to participate in the trustees' board, but would be entitled to representation on an advisory committee.

· To initiate the establishment of an association, the community at large would be invited to acquire memberships.

The two main advantages to this change in governance were outlined for the city of Alliance by members of city council and new mayor, Sam Kirkland. The first, and most important advantage in changing the governance structure was in the way the hospital was financed: the only way the city could finance the hospital was through bonds. The citizens of the city of Alliance were quite through with paying for the hospital, as had been made evident by the failure of several recent bond measures to pass. According to Kirkland, the hospital had not been improved in over 15 years and was "suffering quite markedly." The second reason for changing the structure of the hospital governance was to avoid the constantly changing political winds that seemed to inevitably follow a new city administration.

The plan soon became a topic for debate

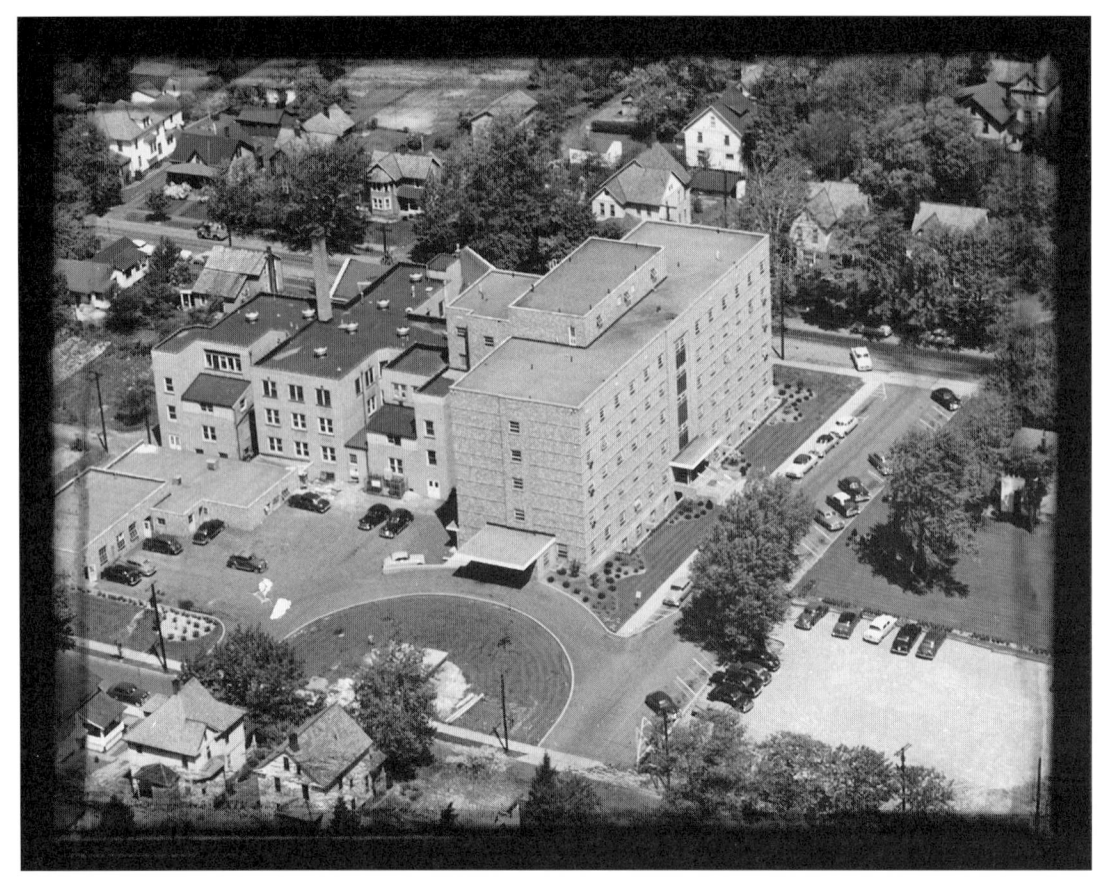

[AERIAL VIEW OF ALLIANCE CITY HOSPITAL · 1953]

within the pages of the *Review*. Immediately following the news of the plan, the Lions Club issued a statement of endorsement for the new structure.[152] The next day, the Alliance Typographical Union "adopted a resolution opposing the proposed relinquishing of control of the Alliance City Hospital by municipal authorities to an association."[153] The sentiment in the town was not unanimous. In a letter to the editor dated 5 March 1945, Mr. Guy Allott writes that

> *A serious depression like that of 1932-53 would compel the hospital to 'fold up' if privately financed just as many private hospitals did in the days of the 30's. The Nurses' Training School would be thrown out in a pinch. The wealth and capital of the city itself is required to maintain such an institution in times of stress.*[154]

The "endorsement war" continued as the hospital plan was endorsed by the Rotary, the American Legion and the Legion Women's' Auxiliary, the Daughters of the Union Veterans of the Civil War, the Sons of the Union Veterans of the Civil War, the Doctors' Wives' Club and finally, on April 12, by the *Alliance*

Review.[155] In an unsigned editorial, the *Review* claimed that the plan was "well matured" and that the plan "had much merit." The editorial went on to claim that

> *We believe ... that a necessary fund with which to meet all the contemplated improvements will be met. It is encouraging to know that a large sum of money for that purpose is now in escrow and that it will be added to in "cold cash" as the time for beginning actual work is launched. It is a forward step and will be one of our larger post-war projects. Everyone realizes the necessity of making possible the improvement of our present institution to give Alliance a bigger and better Hospital.*[156]

Not everyone in Alliance, however, approved of the move; the aforementioned Mr. Allot published no fewer than four letters to the editor in one month, followed closely by Mr. W.H. Wilhelm's three letters during March and April. Those who were against the move made the very persuasive argument that the city was giving away the hospital that the citizens had paid for, and that the hospital had in fact been run very well by the city.[157]

By early April *The Alliance Review* was reporting that city organizations were endorsing the plan by a three-to-one margin. Other groups to come out in favor of the plan included the Elks, the Alliance Women's Club, the City Hospital Auxiliary and the Junior Order of United American Mechanics.

Beginning on April 2, 1945, the *Review* ran a multi-part series about the hospital. The first article was about the now famous study that called for changing the governance (the committee that drew up the plan consisted of F.K. Donaldson, M.E. Rhue, and H.E. Fennerty, with the assistance of hospital expert, Dr. Robin Buerki, of Philadelphia). The *Review* gives a nice summary of the issues surrounding the hospital's "problems" and what might be done to "solve" them[158]:

· The present building was erected in 1918, with a large addition made in 1920. Originally built for 64 beds, it has been readjusted to accommodate about 100 beds.

· The entire service area, which is in the basement, is hampered by an extremely low ceiling, rendering it unattractive and poorly-lighted and ventilated.

· All heating and plumbing facilities are obsolete.

· The building was planned for an efficient operating unit and no provisions whatever were made for expansion. (For instance, if a forty-bed maternity ward were now to be added, the heating, refrigerating, and kitchen facilities could not possibly be expanded to meet new conditions).

· Before any change is made in the present condition of the hospital, the city should be certain that adequate funds so vitally

[ACH Cafeteria · 1953]

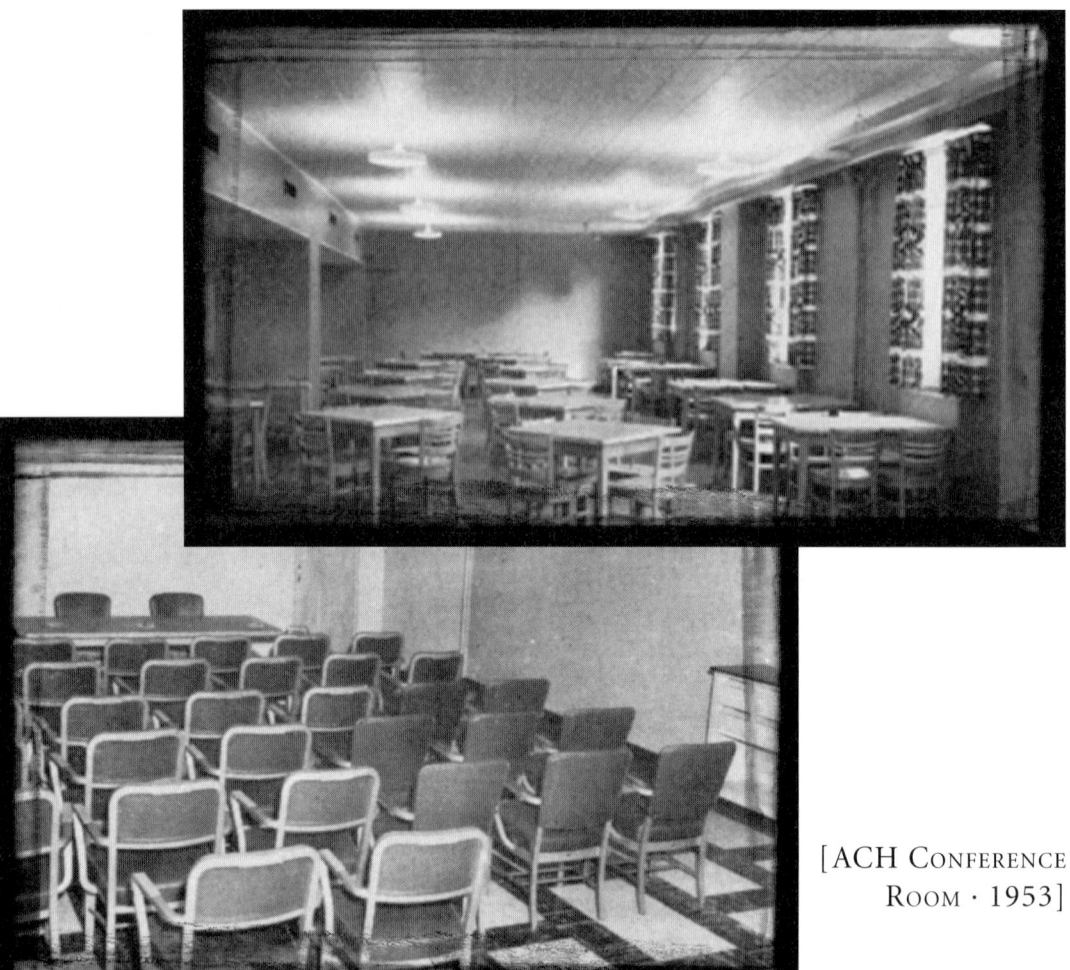

[ACH Conference Room · 1953]

needed will be available for the rehabilitation of the building and equipment.

· That every effort be made to convince the board of the Community Chest the hospital should receive a substantial share of the funds collected.

· That the city of Alliance place in its annual budget a sum sufficient to meet the cost of hospitalization for its indigent.

· If a trained administrator is appointed, he should be given complete authority for the administration of the hospital, and that those groups who have been forced to assume of the administration responsibilities in the past should realize the value of relinquishing those duties to him.

· That the future of the city of Alliance hospital give serious consideration to the establishment of a combined five-year course in conjunction with Mount Union College leading to a Bachelor of Science Degree.

· In any plans that look toward the expansion of the physical plant, each department should be studied so that its needs for additional space may be met.

· The arrangement which allows people who are not in sterile uniforms in the corridor off of an operating room or delivery room is not good practice and should be corrected in any plans for the future.

· Full-time pharmacist, radiologist, pathologist, dentist and nurse anesthetists [sic] be hired.

· The delivery room be used only for deliveries!

In an attempt to counter the obvious bias of the *Review*'s multi-part article about the hospital and to "set the record straight", Mr. Allott started taking out advertisements in the *Review,* thus upping the already high level of argument about the hospital's proposal. A sampling from his advertisements from March-May of 1945:

> · "*Alliance City Hospital was fortunate in having capable, well qualified citizens serve as building commission. Their devotion guaranteed better results than can be expected from a committee of club members who are popular enough to get the votes in this new organization.*"
>
> · "*The evidence does not support any claim of removing 'politics' from the control of this city institution. Rather the contrary. They want to get a control which cannot be upset even following poor management.*"
>
> · "*Veteran hospital employees, who have spent years building up State Retirement insurance have no love for city councilmen, who will vote them off the city payroll — thus taking away their rights for substantial state insurance.*"

Mr. Allott's letters and advertisements seemed to do little to sway the public as the hospital's reorganization moved on through the various committees and voting bodies that needed to approve the changes. On June 17, city council voted 6-1 (the only dissent came from third ward councilman, Nick Trombitas) to approve a lease arrangement with the hospital association, thus clearing the way to move towards a trusteeship arrangement.[159]

Before the final vote, however, a few more voices were to be heard. Letters to the editor from Mr. Harley Ewing and several members of the hospital attacking Mr. Allott's arguments were published in late May.

An interesting shot in the war of letters and advertisements was fired by Mayor Sam Kirkland in a paid advertisement entitled "An Open Letter to the People of Alliance." In his advertisement, Mr. Kirkland writes:

> *There has been a great amount of discussion in recent weeks regarding the proposal*

to lease the Alliance City Hospital to a non-profit association. This is an encouraging situation, for hospital progress depends upon interest — a quantity which has been sorely lacking in Alliance for many years. . . . The Alliance City Hospital has served this community well in the past, but the demands upon the institution have grown. Its operation has become more scientific in nature and complex. There is no fair comparison with operation of a hospital now as against 25 or 30 years ago. . . . I am appealing to the people of Alliance, not to become divided on this hospital question, but get together some plan, and give Alliance a hospital that is second to none. There is no second best in hospitals.[160]

The mayor's advertisement/letter announced an open season for discussion of the hospital governance. On July 18, the *Review* published an advertisement from Mr. W.H. Wilhelm announcing his candidacy for mayor, running on a single issue platform: "I am opposed to leasing the Hospital to any association or clique."[161] At the same time, Mr. Allott and Councilman Trombitas were starting a petition drive to have the decision about the hospital governance turned over to the citizens of Alliance for a vote in the November 1945 general election.

It must have seemed anticlimactic when, in November, the move to trusteeship was approved by the citizens of Alliance by a margin of nearly 80% (6,240 to 1,388). The only thing standing in the way of the hospital's new governance structure at this point was the need to prove that it could raise money — and so immediately, a $100,000 fund drive was started.[162]

The rest of the decade was one long attempt at fundraising. At various times, fund drives in the amount of $70,000, $100,000, and $300,000 were started. The most significant fund drive was the $300,000 "canvas" attempt led by several local businessmen. Chairman Edgar Turkle called it "The greatest community effort in the history of the Alliance area. Never has this community faced as great a challenge as it faces tonight. Never before have we attempted a task of this size and scope."[163] More than 250 local business leaders and workers were planning a complete canvas of Alliance and outlying rural areas. In his speech to the gathered members at the Canvas Kick-Off, held at Mount Union College's Memorial Hall, the Rev. Herbert White told the assembly that "You are not required to give … what you do not have; but you are expected to share in proportion as you are able." The news for this fund drive, unlike drives in the past, was good. Within days after the drive started, the Women's Auxiliary pledged $10,000, the Jaycees $500, and the Alliance Garden Club $500.

Along with the fundraising came early planning for an expansion of the hospital to the

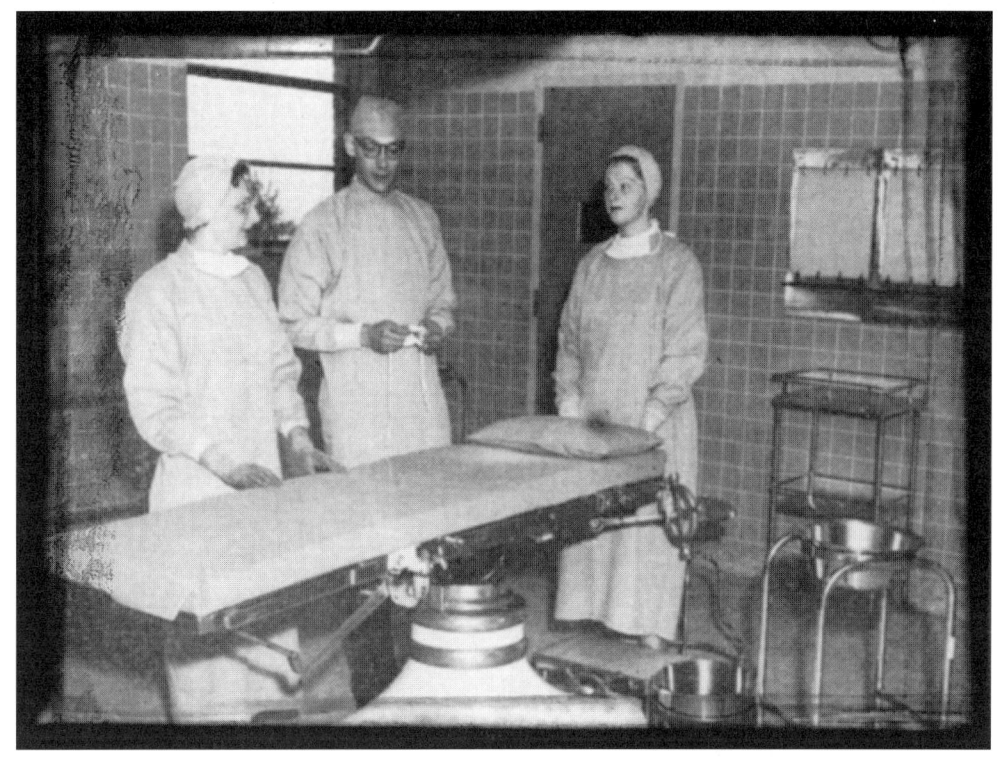

[ACH Surgery · 1953]

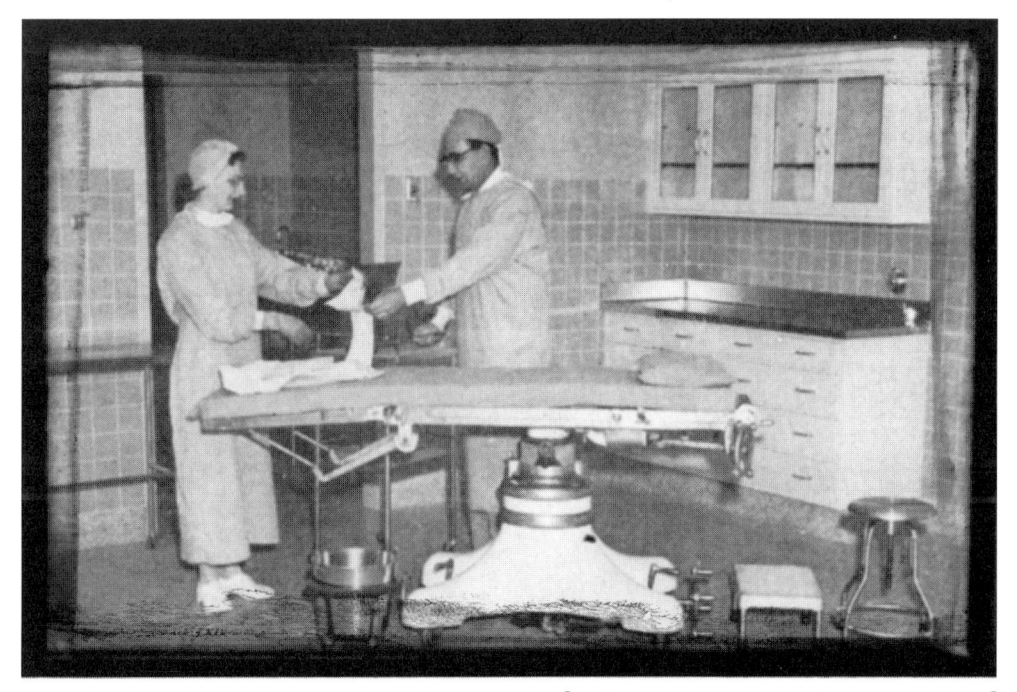

[ACH Emergency Center · 1953]

A CENTURY OF CARING *1940—Present* · 67

east. At a meeting in early 1947, a committee made up of Raymond Wallace, John Caskey, H.L. Weaver, H. Gordon Robertson, J.M. Badertscher, W.H. Metz, and W.U. Phaeffli met with Edgar Turkle to hear about the hospital's plans. According to Turkle, "the new building ... will not quite reach the present 15-foot alley next to the present nurses' home; but that space will be necessary to provide a wider street and parking facilities. The two contiguous properties and two on Rice Street are needed for future expansion."[164]

The "Citizens Hospital Association" took out a number of advertisements in the *Review* to help with the crucial fund drive. The advertisements were models of rhetorical effectiveness. The struggle for the funds was, according to the advertisement, a struggle of life against death. One of the advertisements states, for instance, that "When precious lives are at stake, dollars mean very little. Your hospital faces a crisis. It urgently needs your dollars."[165]

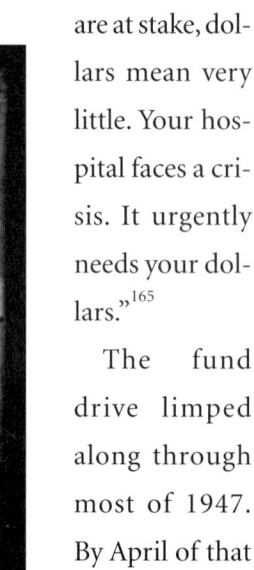

The fund drive limped along through most of 1947. By April of that year it was still $150,000 short despite donations from the city Fire Fighters, the Moose Lodge, the First Methodist Church Women's Society of Christian Service, Mrs. Frank Dussel, the Central Labor Union, the V.F.W., Union Avenue Methodist Church Women's Society of Christian Service, Elks Auxiliary, St. Paul's Lutheran Church, the Rotary Club, the Lions Club, Daughters of Union Veterans, and the Women's division of the Chamber of Commerce.

By the end of the year, however, fund drive chairman, Edgar Turkle, was planning a victory dinner—despite a slow start, the drive gained extraordinary momentum, bringing in

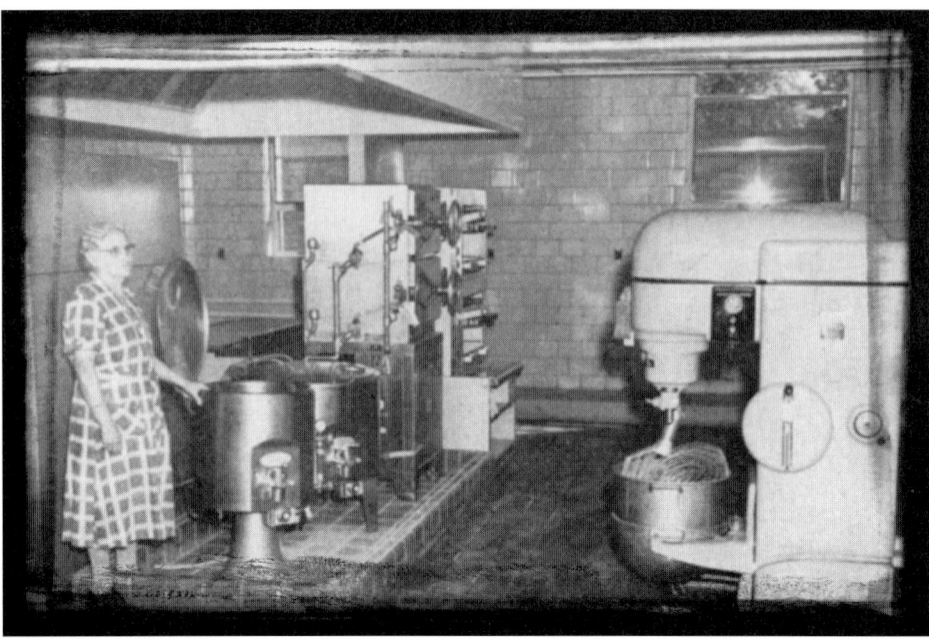

[ACH Kitchen · 1953]

close to $100,000 in one weekend, spurred on by the city of Sebring's generous contribution of $35,800.[166] The drive was put over the top by a gift of $10,000 by Alliance Lodge 467 B.P.O. Elks in what was called the "largest single contribution in a community enterprise in the history of Alliance."[167]

Finally, on Tuesday, February 10, 1948, a celebration dinner was planned at the Alliance Country Club to celebrate the "splendid cooperation in the solicitation of nearly 3,000 pledges in the Hospital Canvas which is nearing completion."[168]

And then the triumph: on Wednesday, February 11, 1948, the *Alliance Review* announced that a total of $315,120.50 had been raised and that the addition would indeed be built. The Rev. White remarked that "This is no one person's victory . . . it is the victory of all the citizens of the greater Alliance area who saw a challenge and accepted it."[169] It was reported that the "extra" $15,000 would be used to build a new nurses' dormitory.

The only remaining order of business in the transition from city management to a trusteeship was to hold the first election of trustees. Anyone who had given $5 or more was eligible to vote. The election was slated to occur on Friday, March 19, 1948. The first trustee elected was Harry Wheeler who would represent city council. The remaining 10 trustees elected at the March meeting were as follows: Mrs. Karl Fiegenschuh, William Metz, Harold Hubbard, William Anderson, Raymond Wallace, Willis Biery, Spencer Sebrell, H. Gordon Robertson, John Liber, and P.R. Ickes. Also

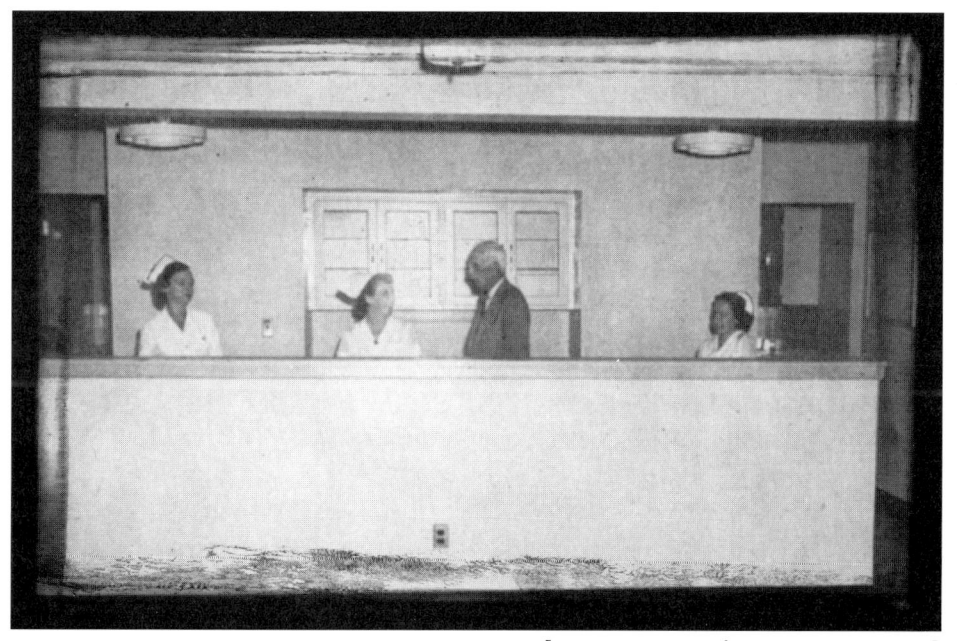

[ACH NURSES' STATION · 1953]

on the board would be Mayor Althouse and Edgar Turkle, who was elected president in a unanimous vote.

After the elections it was back to business as usual for the hospital. A new director of the school of nursing was hired, Ms. Lula Bell Herold of Pittsburgh, and the various business and staffing concerns that cropped up during the transfer of power were worked out.[170]

The decade ended on a sad note with the passing of Dr. Perry King, who had been on the staff of the hospital since 1906. Dr. King, often called the "dean of practicing physician-surgeons" was felled by a heart attack after returning from a trip to California. A member of the Mount Union College class of 1899, King had been chief of staff at the hospital for more than twenty-five years, and had been volunteer physician for Mount Union College's athletic teams for more than forty years.[171]

Towards the beginning of the process of building the new addition, a small news item that appeared in the Canton *Repository*, would prove to have big repercussions for the Alliance Hospital. According to the *Repository*, the hospital was eligible for federal aid (something many in Alliance had hoped for); accordingly, planning for the new addition was quickly completed and building was scheduled to begin on November 15, 1948. The project was now being called the "million-dollar hospital" by both the *Repository* and Edgar Turkle, President of the Board of Trustees. Plans were in the works for a 165-bed hospital to be financed through a combination of public subscription and bond money. As of the writing of the *Repository* article, $850,000 had been raised by bonds and $100,000 by subscription. The only remaining question was the need to raise an additional $150,000 by the federally imposed deadline of July 1, 1950.

According to a pamphlet published by the hospital advocating for the emergency bond issue, the reasons for having to ask the public for money once again were complicated; according to the pamphlet:

· *Three years ago we proposed and you approved a bond issue for $700,000. That was in May 1947. Then in September 1947, you approved the trustee form of management for the City Hospital at a general election.*

· *In January of 1948, we found that building and equipment costs had risen so sharply, that it was necessary to put on a voluntary campaign for added funds and you, the citizens of Alliance, subscribed more than $300,000.*

· *In the fall of 1949, the Division of Hospital Facilities, Ohio State Board of Health, finally put its stamp of approval on the architect's plans, calling for a $1,575,000 hospital based upon per capita needs of our constantly growing community.*

· *Where was this sum to come from? . . .*

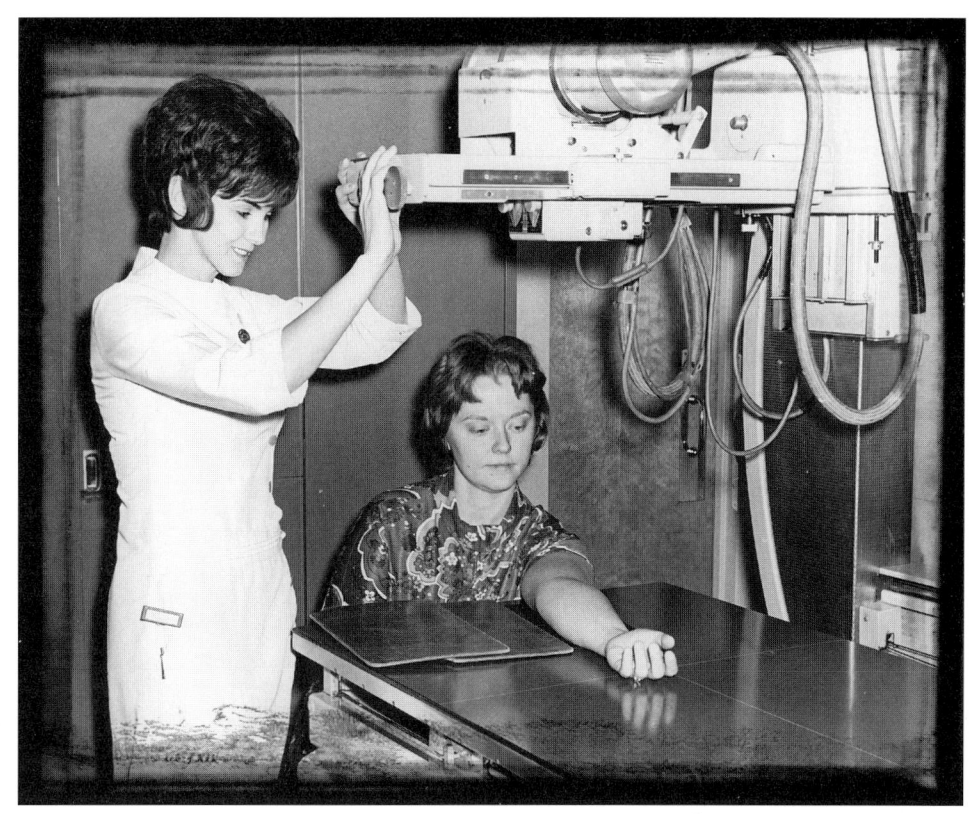

[ACH X-Ray · 1972]

There was only one answer. From the $900,000 on hand, from $150,000 to be raised by another bond issue and from matching federal funds of $525,000.[172]

Much of the information about the new addition and the necessary bond issue comes from advertisements the Hospital Association took out in the *Alliance Review* during the crucial months leading up to the vote. A February 16 advertisement spells out the hospital's argument when it claims

The new hospital will consist of six floors in all with ground level devoted to pharmacy room, kitchen, storage, a conference room as health information center, and cafeteria.

First floor will have lobby and offices, hospitality shop, soda fountain, records room, and doctor's library. Emergency suite at south will have two emergency rooms, recovery room, autopsy room, private corridor and elevator.

Second, third, and fourth floors will be devoted to medical and surgical general patient care. Lavatory facilities and clothes closets in every room. A patient solarium on every floor, no room with more than four beds as well as two-bed and private rooms.

Fifth floor devoted to surgery, which will include major surgeries, eye, ear, nose and

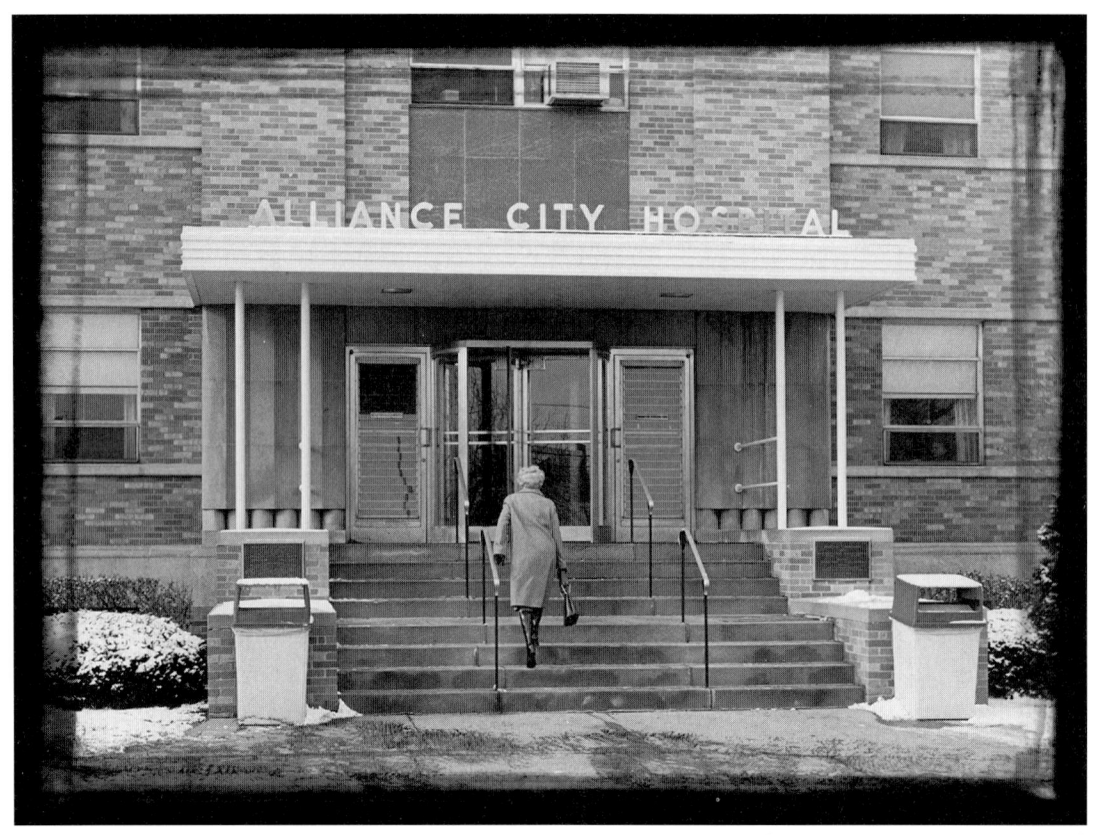

[ACH Entrance · 1972]

throat surgery, oral and dental surgery and four recovery beds.

Ground level of present building will be converted to out-patient clinic, locker rooms, sewing and housekeeper's rooms and this section will be connected to the laundry.

First floor of present building will be given over to radiology, pathology, and physical therapy with facilities for the Board of Health including visiting nurses, city food inspection and city health department.

The second floor will be the maternity suite with twenty-eight nursing beds, four labor beds and twenty-eight long term bassinets.

The third floor will be devoted to pediatrics with provision for a resident physician.

At the south will be the new laundry which will mean an annual savings of approximately $8,000.

On October 4, 1950, the *Alliance Review* was able to report that the hospital had the "go ahead" to start receiving bids for the new addition, now priced at $1.5 million dollars. The architects, Kling and Frost of Youngstown,

[ACH Snack Shop · 1972]

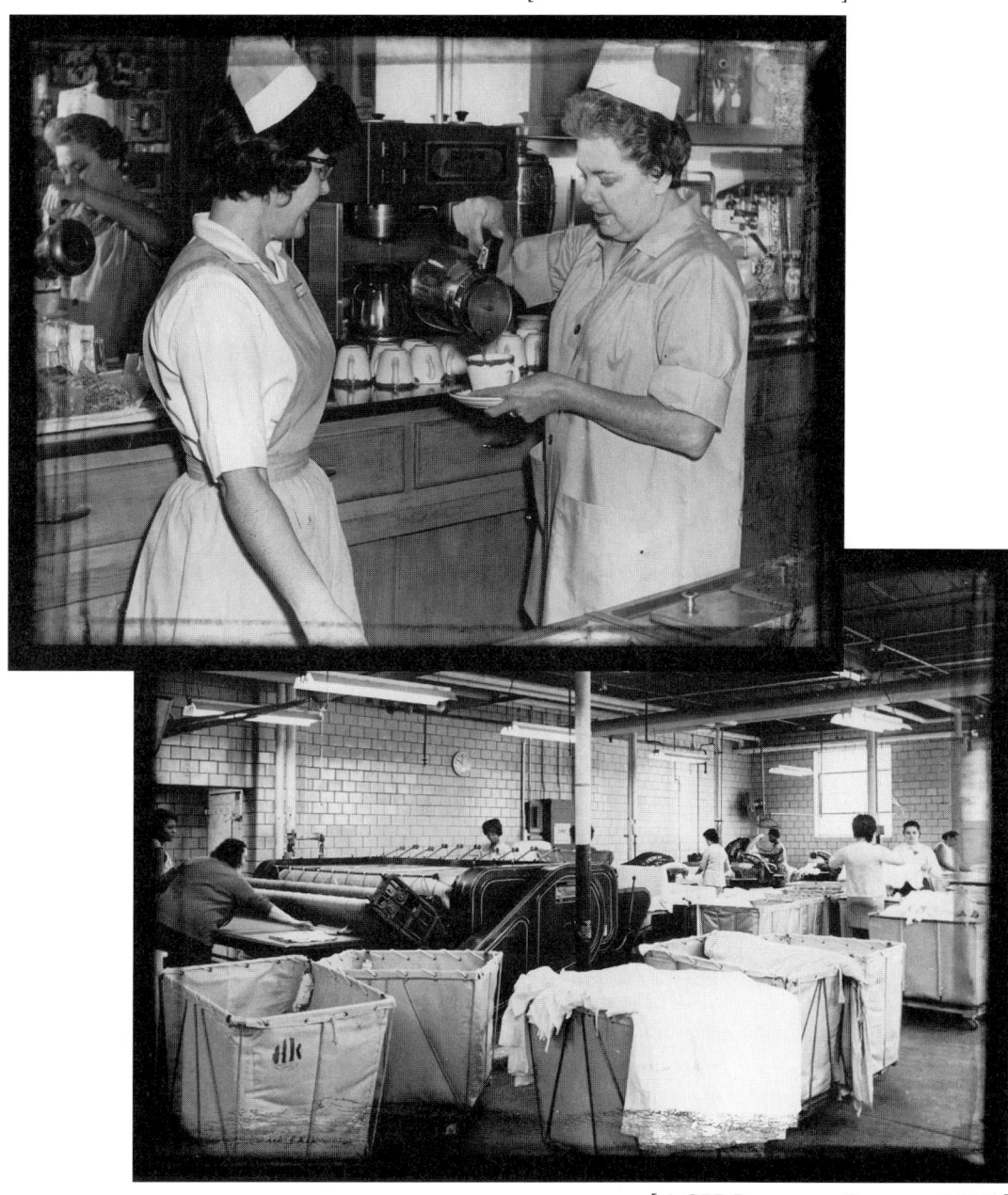

[ACH Laundry Room · 1972]

created several alternatives for the hospital depending upon the costs. According to Otto Kling, "one alternate will call for a new hospital building, but omitting the fourth floor. The other asks bids on a new building, but omitting the west wing of a proposed fifth floor."[173] Kling and Frost planned on starting the bidding process in November 1950.

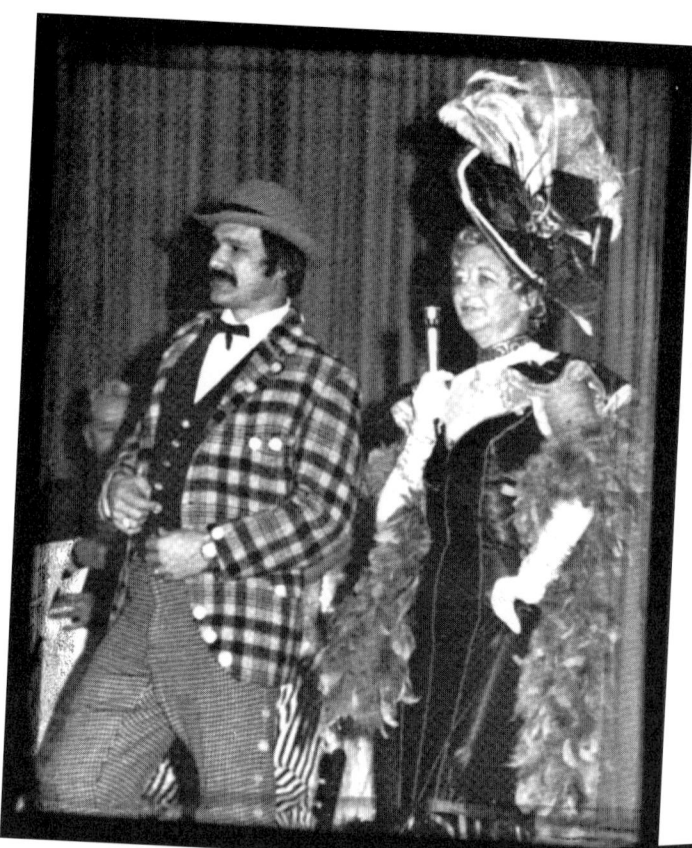

In November, the Alliance construction firm of Paul A. Kintz placed the lowest bid for a 105-bed addition "along with the laundry and boiler plant at a cost of $722,068."[174] Plumbing and heating contracts went to the Spohm Heating and Ventilating Company of Cleveland whose bid was $257,905. According to the *Review*, the estimate for the entire cost of the addition was $1,305,204, which would leave more than $130,000 in a contingency fund for any cost overruns or

[FRACTURED FOLLIES · 1976]

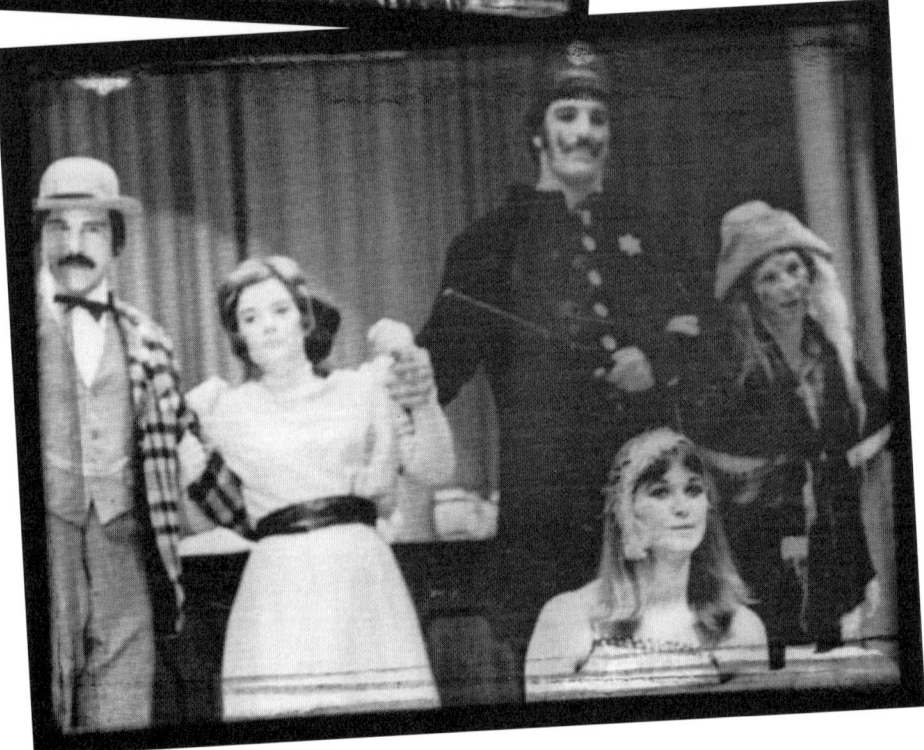

would be used for repairs and renovations on the old hospital building.

The funding for the new building broke down as follows:

- More than $1,000,000 was raised through membership subscriptions and two successful bond issues.
- $525,000 came from federal assistance.
- The state of Ohio came through with a donation of $25,000.

As soon as the funds were raised for the new addition, the members of the hospital board turned their attention towards the renovation of the old hospital building. According to the Board Chairman, Edgar Turkle, even "when the new units are completed, Alliance will lack a complete modern hospital unless the old institution is remodeled."[175] At a meeting held in the Mount Union College library, Mayor Harley Ewing named a fundraising commission to look for the additional money necessary for the repairs. The committee consisted of Dr. Robert King of the hospital staff; Mrs. J. J. Hurst of the Women's Auxiliary; Dr. D.W. Morgan of City Council; and Clarence Steffy of the *Review*. The new addition was finished in 1954 and the "old" hospital building was remodeled and dedicated in 1956.

During this time of change, another event happened very quietly that signaled the end of an era for the hospital. According to the December 10, 1949 issue of the *Alliance Review*, "quietly and without fanfare, one of Alliance's landmarks" was coming down: the Whitacre home, which had been the location of the original Deaconess home and hospital, was being razed.[176] The article gives no real information about why the home was razed except to note that the nurses were now housed in the "old Judd property" at 1717 South Arch Ave. According to internal documents, the nursing school was closed in 1949 after graduating a class of seven.[177]

In 1953, as the hospital stood on the precipice of the modern age, Robert B. Carey was employed as the hospital's administrator. The Chief of Surgery was Dr. L.F. Mutschmann, Chief of Medicine was Dr. W.E. Elliott, Business Manager was Herman Wright, and the Director of Nursing was Mrs. Hazel Peebles. At this point in the hospital's history there were thirty-nine physicians, eighteen dentists, and ten other officers on the staff. The officers of the medical staff were President, Dr. J.L. McClinock; Secretary, Dr. J.J. Thomas; and Treasurer, Dr. H.L. Weaver. The Women's Auxiliary was coordinated by Mrs. Guy Hoover, Mrs. J.L. Harvey, Mrs. Donald Peterson, and Mrs. W.G. Robertson.

This same year saw the start of the Auxiliary's Memorial Fund which over the years has helped to fund an electrocardiograph machine, a pressure gradient machine, electric candles for the chapel, art work for the hospital, and the bronze leader board for the lobby.[178] 1953 also saw the start of the Auxiliary service shop, the antecedent to the snack and gift shops.[179]

According to the hospital's own records, at this time (1953-56) several members of the hospital staff who would become well known for their work with the city of Alliance joined the staff. These included Dr. Delmar Gard (who later had a Pediatric/Children's ward named after him); Floyd Spurgeon, longtime physical therapist, and Mrs. W.G. Yanney, the longtime administrator's assistant. Many of the doctors who were on staff at this moment (1956) were still on staff in 1979, when the last history of the hospital was written, providing, in the words of said history, "a remarkable continuity of service."

In 1956, the Carey administration published the hospital's economic forecast and explained to the citizens of Alliance how the hospital's budget was organized. According to Carey, 64% of hospital funds went to salaries and wages, 21% to medical supplies and equipment, 5% to pharmaceuticals, 4% to utilities, 3% to insurance, and 3% to food. Carey made some attempts to fund various improvements that were largely failures, including a bond issue that was voted down by the citizens of Alliance in 1960. In that same year, however, the business manager of the *Alliance Review*, Mr. Paul Siddall, led a fundraising effort which netted the hospital over $250,000.

According to the 1959 *Annual Report*, the hospital was serving the city of Alliance and surrounding areas to full capacity. During the year 1959 the hospital did 131,689 laboratory examinations, performed 2,195 operations, saw 9,831 emergency room patients, delivered 1,252 babies, gave 1,021 blood transfusions, served 208,344 meals, did 922,875 pounds of laundry, and cared for 7,228 patients. During this year, the hospital averaged 78% occupancy overall, and 59% in the maternity ward, 53% in pediatrics and 89% in the surgical units. During the same time the hospital incurred $959,735 in labor costs, had $406,239 in operating expenses, and spent $11,532 on capital improvements.

In 1971, Robert Carman became the hospital's administrator. Carman was instrumental in many improvements and changes in the hospital. Under the Carman administration, the personnel handbook was updated and a helicopter was used for the first time to transport patients to and from the hospital in emergencies.

Also during the Carman administration, a comprehensive chaplaincy program was created with the help of the Alliance Ministers' Association, which signed up clergymen for visitation for a week at a time, three days a week.

The biggest event of the Carman administration was a $4,000,000 building campaign to provide room for physical therapy, radiology, emergency, new laboratories, a new

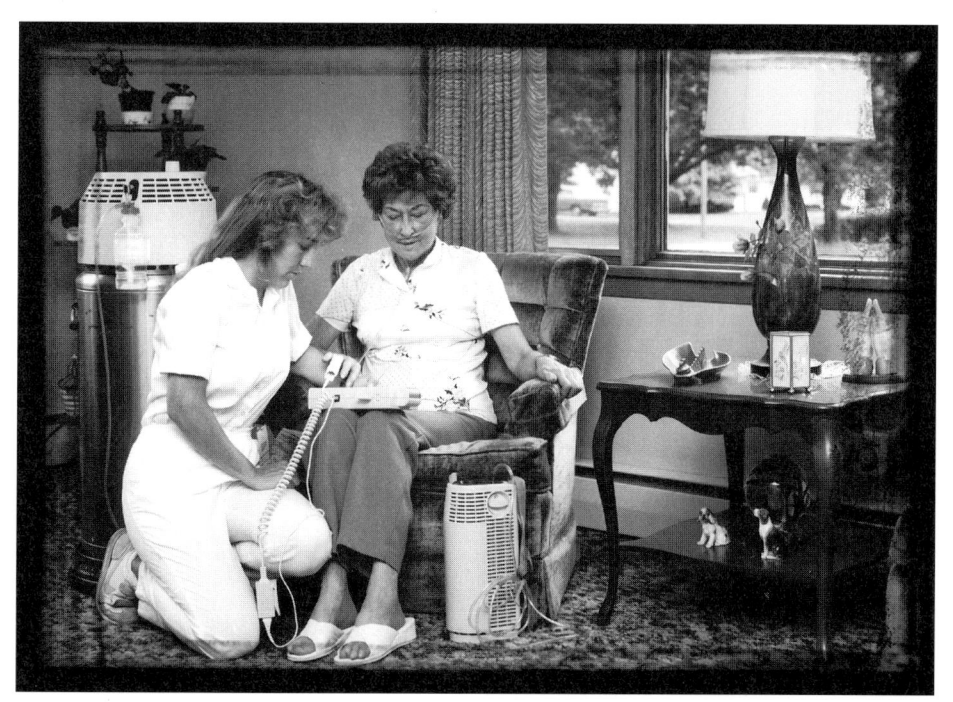

[ACH VISITING NURSE · 1985]

chapel, a snack bar, new lobby space, and new parking. Most of the money for the new building (over $3,000,000) was raised through a public bond to be paid off over 25 years.

Work on the 54,000 square foot addition began in September 1974 and was completed in July 1976. The completed structure contained waiting and admitting areas, a snack bar, gift shop, emergency room, outpatient services as well as various laboratories and treatment rooms. This addition saw the emergency room entrance move to E. College Street where it remained until 1997.

The new addition to the hospital grew out of a master plan created in 1970 by the board of hospital trustees and the board of hospital commissioners. One of the key facts of this master plan was the number of residents the hospital served in the area (this was figured at roughly ten townships and four counties). Between 1960 and 1970, the number of residents served increased from 92,075 to 100,294.[180]

The addition was funded by the Citizens Hospital Association and ended up costing slightly more than $5,000,000. Most of the financing came through twenty-year bonds, although more than $450,000 came from individual and corporate donations including the Timken, Hoover, and Stark Foundations, the hospital's medical staff, and the trustees. Along with the new building came almost $400,000 worth of new equipment, including new radiology machines. According to hospital administrator Carman,

Completion of the Alliance City Hospital Modernization and Expansion Program is but the beginning of a new era in the Hospital's ability to better serve its patients. This addition is truly a tribute to the many people of Alliance who have devoted count-

[ACH Pharmacy · 1985]

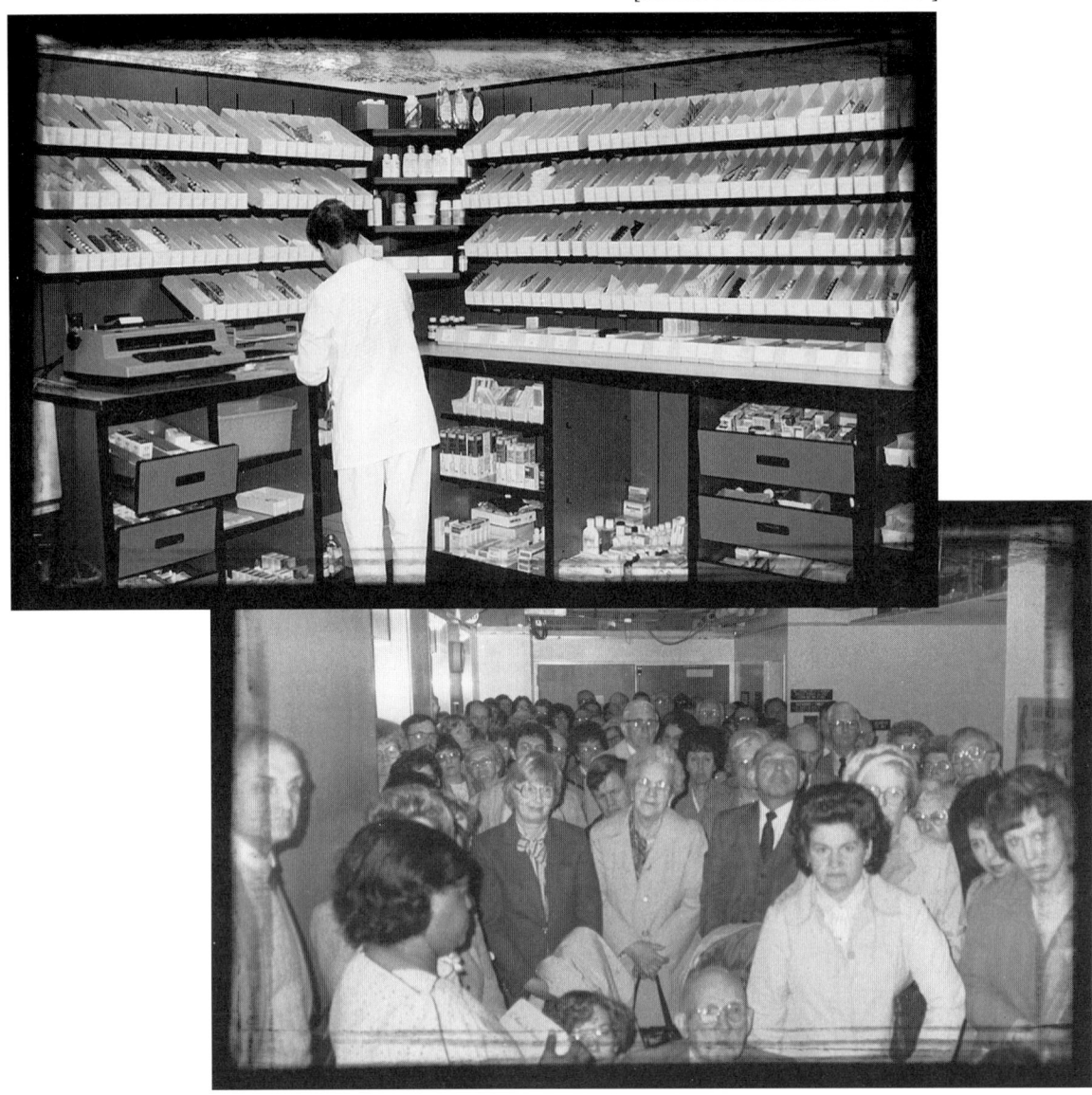

[ACH Open House (Surgery) · 1985]

less hours of their time and service to this project.

Two other needs at this time were a new parking lot (one was eventually built on the corner of Arch and Rice Streets) and a "Medical Arts Building" for physicians and others to use as office space. Eventually, the old Kroger building on State Street became such a facility. According to the *Review*, the hospital wanted to buy the building and its property for roughly $200,000 and divide the space into at least ten offices.[181]

The biggest nonphysical plant change to come to the hospital at this time (1975-6), other than a 9% increase in rates, was the decision by the hospital to allow fathers into the delivery room during natural childbirth. According to Mrs. Charles Hanks, the hospital had made this move because the national trends in childbirth were towards the "natural style" and that "facilities should be made available for those who choose that way."[182]

In 1975, the hospital celebrated its 75th anniversary in very low-key manner. The addition was half done and there is little mention in either the *Annual Report* or the *Alliance Review* of any sort of celebration. According to the *Review*, the hospital marked its anniversary with a small reception of employees and invited guests that featured a cake-cutting, musical selections by Alliance pianist, Hans Lang, and the presentation of a special historical scroll to each employee and patient.

Around this same time, a series of letters appeared in the *Alliance Review* regarding the quality of care at the hospital. Mrs. Charles Standing of W. Ely Street in Alliance wrote a nice letter to the *Review* that said, in part,

> *I believe the 75th Anniversary of the Alliance City Hospital is an ideal time to make the people of Alliance fully aware of how very fortunate we are to have such an excellent hospital in our city. In Sept. of 1975 I was a patient in Alliance City Hospital and because of personal complications I was transferred to a Cleveland Hospital. . . . So I am writing from experience and not hearsay. The rooms, service, care, meals, etc. are far superior here in Alliance compared to the Cleveland Hospital and at a fraction of the cost.*[183]

November 1975, brought the retirement of Dr. Robert King, the second in a long line of Kings who had served the hospital (Dr. King's father had been Dr. Perry King, former Chief-of-Staff). A native of Alliance and graduate of Alliance High School and Mount Union College, Dr. King had worked at the hospital for more than thirty-two years. He received his medical degree from Harvard University and had done residencies at Bellevue and Roosevelt hospitals in New York City. He returned to Alliance in January 1943, to set up a surgical practice. In an interesting side note, Dr. King's wife was the former Peggy Perkins, daughter of the famous Maxwell Perkins, an editor at Scribner's Press in New York whose editorial work with Thomas Wolfe, William Faulkner, and Ernest Hemingway, to name just a few, made him the most sought after editor in the country. One of their sons, the actor Perry King, appeared in several television series including *Melrose Place* and *Riptide* as well as over 40 films including *Mandingo* and *The Lords of Flatbush*. Another son, Max, was city editor for the *Philadelphia Inquirer*.

The big news in 1976, other than the opening of the new addition, was a strike by the hospital's nursing staff. On Thursday morning, September 30, the nurses set up picket lines in front of the hospital, protesting the fact that the hospital "has refused to accept any proposals that would improve patient care and raise standards of practice."[184] While much of the strike was about economic matters, the key differences between the nurses and the hospital had to do with items like the establishment of eight-hour shifts, willingness to abide by the American Nurses' Associations Code for Nurses, and the hospital's alleged unwillingness to establish a Nursing Advisory Committee to "provide a method of communication between the nurses and the hospital concerning patient care." The strike lasted ten weeks and was settled in mid-December with a pay raise and full recognition by the hospital of the nurses' union.

In 1978, F. Douglas Wert became the hospital's new administrator. Under his supervision, the hospital made many changes, including:

- the addition of ten new physicians, including specialists in orthopedics as well as thoracic and vascular surgery.
- A project to automate much of the laboratory equipment and the full accreditation of the American College of Pathologists.
- Addition of ultrasound equipment.
- Microsurgical instruments which gave the hospital the ability to do retina repairs as well as work on small vessels in the eye.
- New fetal monitors, pediatric monitoring, and emergency defibrillation equipment was made available throughout the hospital.
- The respiratory therapy department was developed: Certified and registered technicians were hired and the area was able to perform automated pulmonary function tests, micro blood gas analysis, stress tests as well as EKG and EEGs.

At this time the medical staff was headed by Dr. Robert Reed. The Director of Nursing was Mrs. Jane Aral and the Administrative Assistant for Patient Services was Mrs. Joyce Siefke.

As the eighties began, the hospital was again looking towards the future. In January 1981, Jane Aral, the Director of Nursing, was arguing for an increase in the Maximum Care Unit.[185] This need had been determined by a "community needs assessment" which had been undertaken by the hospital in late 1980. The assessment found that oftentimes patients had to be moved out of the Maximum Care area and into the hallway or other wards when more critical patients needed help. Of primary concern to many at the hospital was the fact that even though the hospital had added a new building in 1976, the Maximum Care Unit was still in the old 1917 building and was in dire need of updating.

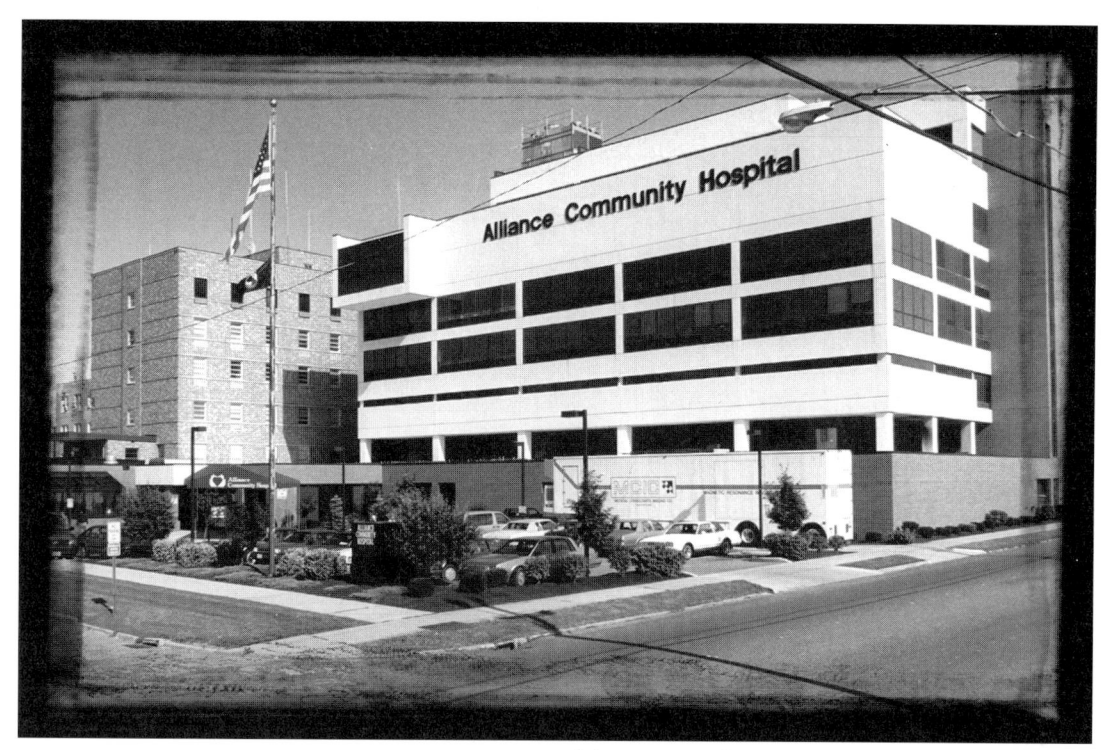

[ALLIANCE COMMUNITY HOSPITAL · 1989]

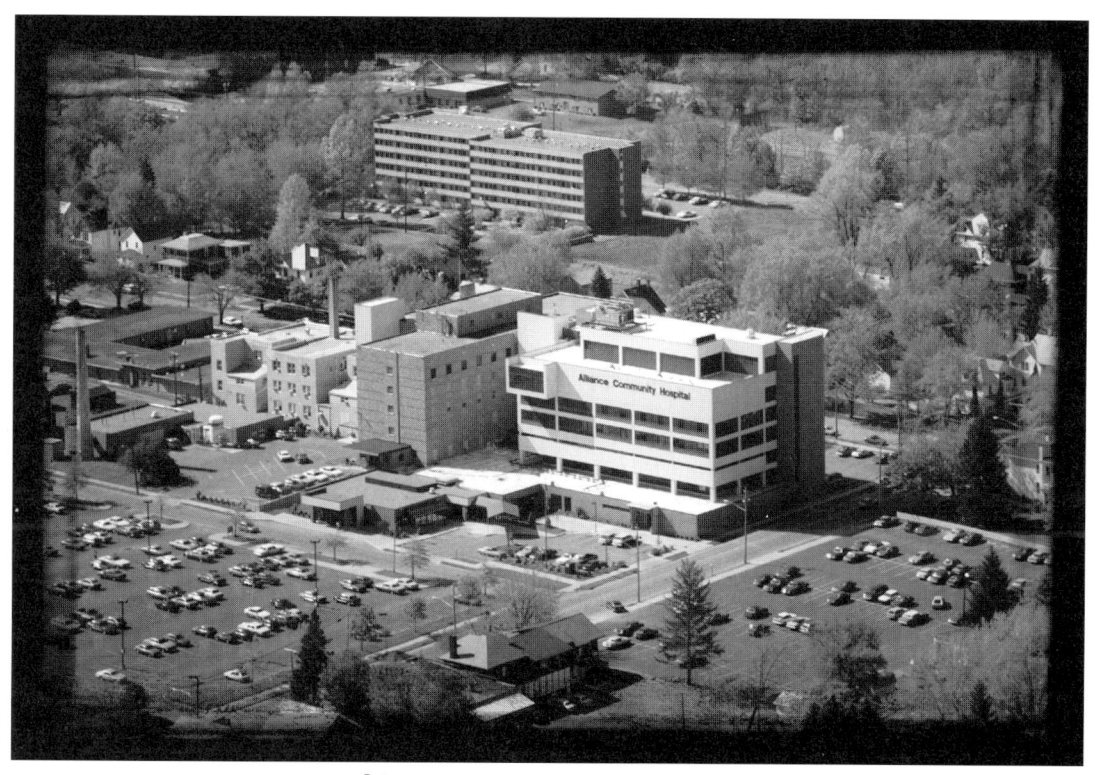

[AERIAL VIEW OF ALLIANCE COMMUNITY HOSPITAL · 1989]

A CENTURY OF CARING   *1940–Present* · 81

In April 1981, the hospital began the process of long-range planning. A committee headed by Dr. James Rodman and Mayor James Puckett worked with a consultant to look at space and staffing needs for the future. The trustees also hired an architect to do site planning for the physical plant.[186] According to the 1981 *Annual Report*,

> *The Planning Committee received a voluminous report from its health care facility consultant, Larry Pugh and Associates, and also a careful market analysis from Cambridge Associates. These studies outlined a need for improvements in our facilities and an architectural firm, Collins & Rimer of Cleveland[,] Ohio was commissioned to create a master plan for the facilities development . . . for the long range future . . . We expect that a plan for a new building will be unveiled in 1982.*

1981 also saw the redecoration of many of the patient rooms and the reorganization of a quality assurance program that included the auditing of each patient's regimen of care. At the beginning of the eighties, the hospital was serving 243,600 meals, cleaning 834,300 pounds of laundry, delivering 700 babies, and performing 4,000 operations per year.

1982 saw the kickoff of what the hospital was calling the "Excellence for the Eighties" campaign, which involved fundraising, new buildings, and an increased emphasis upon hiring and retention of new medical staff. 1982 also saw the opening of the Flower Box shop, the result of a three year program put together and staffed by the members of the Hospital Auxiliary. Fresh flowers, which could be bought in the gift shop, were now arranged by members of the auxiliary, headed by Alma Teeters, Marge Downes, and Ann Wilson.[187]

The planning for a new $6,000,000 addition was continued with the hiring, in November, of the Kintz Construction Company as the construction managers for the new building. The construction plans called for an addition of three floors on top of the 1974 building (this had been planned for in the original 1974 design) and the remodeling of other sections. The new construction would provide a new surgery unit, new obstetrical and pediatrics facilities, and a new maximum care unit. Jack Peters, of Butler-Wick, chairman of the Hospital Associations finance committee, remarked that the work would not be a "fresh expansion but rather a renovation of operations like [the] obstetrical unit which is located in a building built in 1913 [sic]."[188]

In September 1982, Carl Medley was appointed as the hospital's interim Chief Executive Officer. He replaced Douglas Wert, who left suddenly to take a position in Dayton, Ohio.[189] In three short years, Wert had built the hospital's net worth by over $3,700,000 (an increase of roughly 76%). In his farewell to city council, Wert claimed that

> *The quality of work of each department*

has significantly improved, and fine new leadership has been added in many departments. The public image of the hospital, as well as employee morale and self-image, has been enhanced by virtue of a higher standard of quality care and the addition of many new services. . . . These accomplishments are the product of a good team and the work of many in our hospital family, yet I share in the pride of these constructive changes.[190]

During that same month, city council gave tentative approval to $10,000,000 worth of building and rebuilding at the hospital. The money would either be raised by a public sale of bonds by McDonald and Company or a private issuance of bonds by Butler and Wick.[191]

1982 was another in a string of eventful years for the Hospital. In the *Annual Report* for 1982, Carl Medley attempted to sum up all that had happened when he wrote that:

The Board, Administration, and Medical Staff will continue to meet the cost containment and quality of care issues that face the health care industry in general, and specifically Alliance City Hospital, with the goal of "Excellence for the Eighties" always in mind.

The rest of the eighties were about progress. In 1983, E. Richard Moore was hired as the new Administrator/CEO and Mrs. Nancy Tallman was hired as the new director of nursing. In his first *Annual Report*, Mr. Moore wrote that

1983 will be remembered as the year the plans for the 7 million dollar renovation were culminated. This project is the product of 2.5 years of planning to arrive at what the Board of Trustees, hospital management and

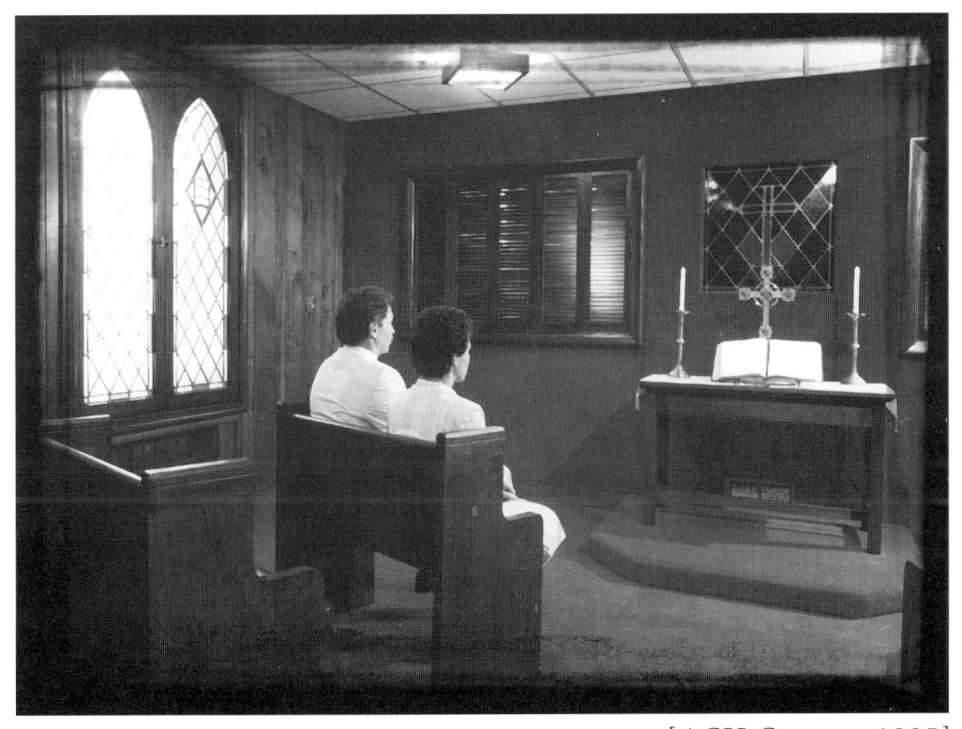

[ACH CHAPEL · 1985]

A CENTURY OF CARING *1940—Present* · 83

physicians agree will provide more effective use of space in order to provide the best possible quality of care.

By the end of 1983 the Fund Balance at the hospital was over $10,000,000 for the first time. In February 1984 the hospital issued improvement bonds in the amount of $4,800,000. This amount, combined with another $4,000,000 to come from the hospital and the city would finance the improvements to the building that Mr. Moore discussed in his letter to the Board.

The renovation project was started in March 1984, and at the time the 1984 *Annual Report* was written, it was 65% complete. The hospital planned to start moving equipment into the new surgical ward in late April of the same year.

The other big changes in 1984 were due to a massive restructuring of the Medicare system. According to Board Chairman Charles Grove, "A new system 38 IBM computer has been installed and placed in operation. This total system change allows Alliance City Hospital to cope with the reimbursement changes."[192]

Medical improvements and changes in 1984 included the acquisition of a computerized axial tomography (CAT) scan machine as well as vast improvements in the area of Cardiac Care. According to Dr. Andres Lao, President of the Medical/Dental staff, these improvements "made the hospital able to provide full critical care services and to do all non-invasive diagnostic cardiology for our patients."

The mid-eighties did see a slight decline in average census, from 135.0 in 1982 to 104.4 in 1984, although very few were worried by this (many cited the increase in outpatient care), a few were beginning to question the hospital's increases in staff and funding. Dr. David Goldman addressed this in his 1983 *Annual Report* by writing that the community of Alliance had shown an "ever-increasing confidence in our institution and its staff," and that Alliance was not to be worried about the decrease in usage (which, according to Goldman, merely reflected the general economics and demographics of the city of Alliance).

In the *Annual Report* for 1985, new Hospital CEO Melvin Pucci could write with some confidence that "The past year proved to be a time of great change for Alliance City Hospital. Significant progress was achieved in improving not only the quality but the availability and cost-effectiveness of vital healthcare services provided to our community." Major events in 1985 included the opening of a new OB section, "The Birth Place," as well as the opening of the Alliance City Hospital Cancer Care Program. Both of these eliminated the need to drive long distances for specialized maternity, pediatric, and oncology services.

1985 also saw the start of a new long-range planning cycle. In January, the Hospital Board adopted a nine-point plan to promote the local health care facility through advertising campaigns; attract physicians; provide a different way of showing the financial health of the institution; and promote the activities level of the hospital.[193]

Perhaps the biggest news of 1985 was the official opening, in March, of the new 13,400 square foot surgical suite, followed closely by the opening, in September, of the new Intensive Care Unit (including pediatric and surgical ICU sections). According to the *Annual Report*,

> *These facilities are a dream come true for thousands of area patients served by the hospital and represent the culmination of four years of careful planning, design, and construction under the supervision of the Board of Trustees, Building Commission, the Planning Committee, physicians, hospital staff and many other interested friends of the hospital.*

The jewel of the addition, the new surgical suite, was now considered by the staff to be

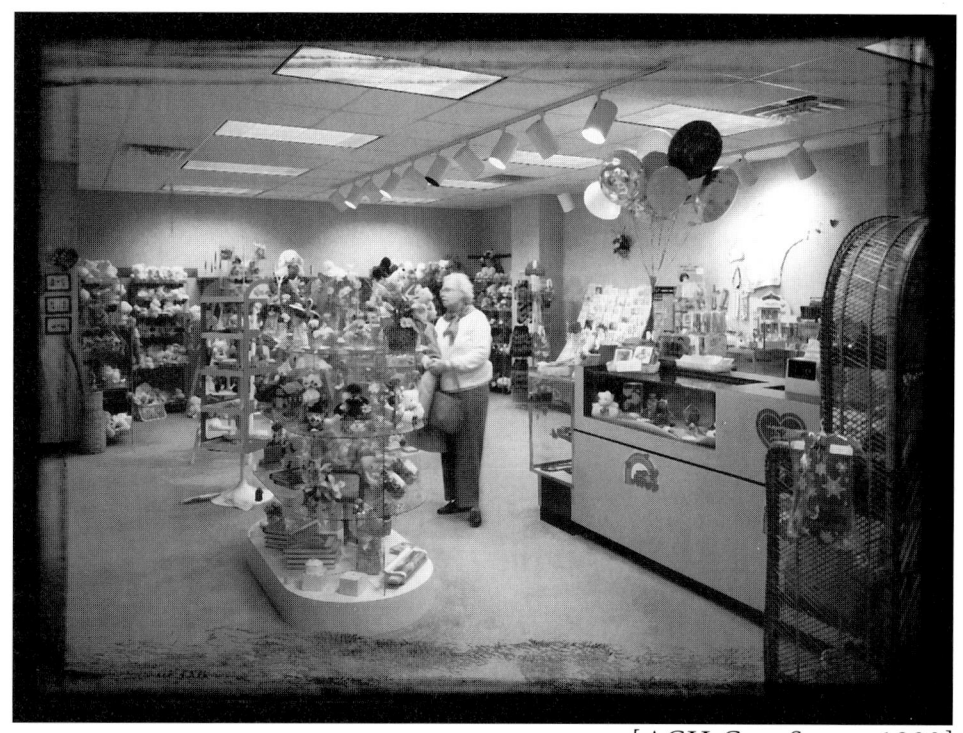

[ACH GIFT SHOP · 1989]

"state-of-the-art in every respect." The suite was equipped with "sophisticated communications and environmental-control equipment," and was constructed to have "two operating rooms for general surgery and four for special procedures—eye, orthopedic, endoscopic and cystoscopic."[194] The new ICU contained twelve private, continuously monitored rooms based around the "island concept" where nurses could keep close tabs on those most critically ill patients.

In April, a survey given to hospital management identified several priorities for the

[ACH ICU Room · 1985]

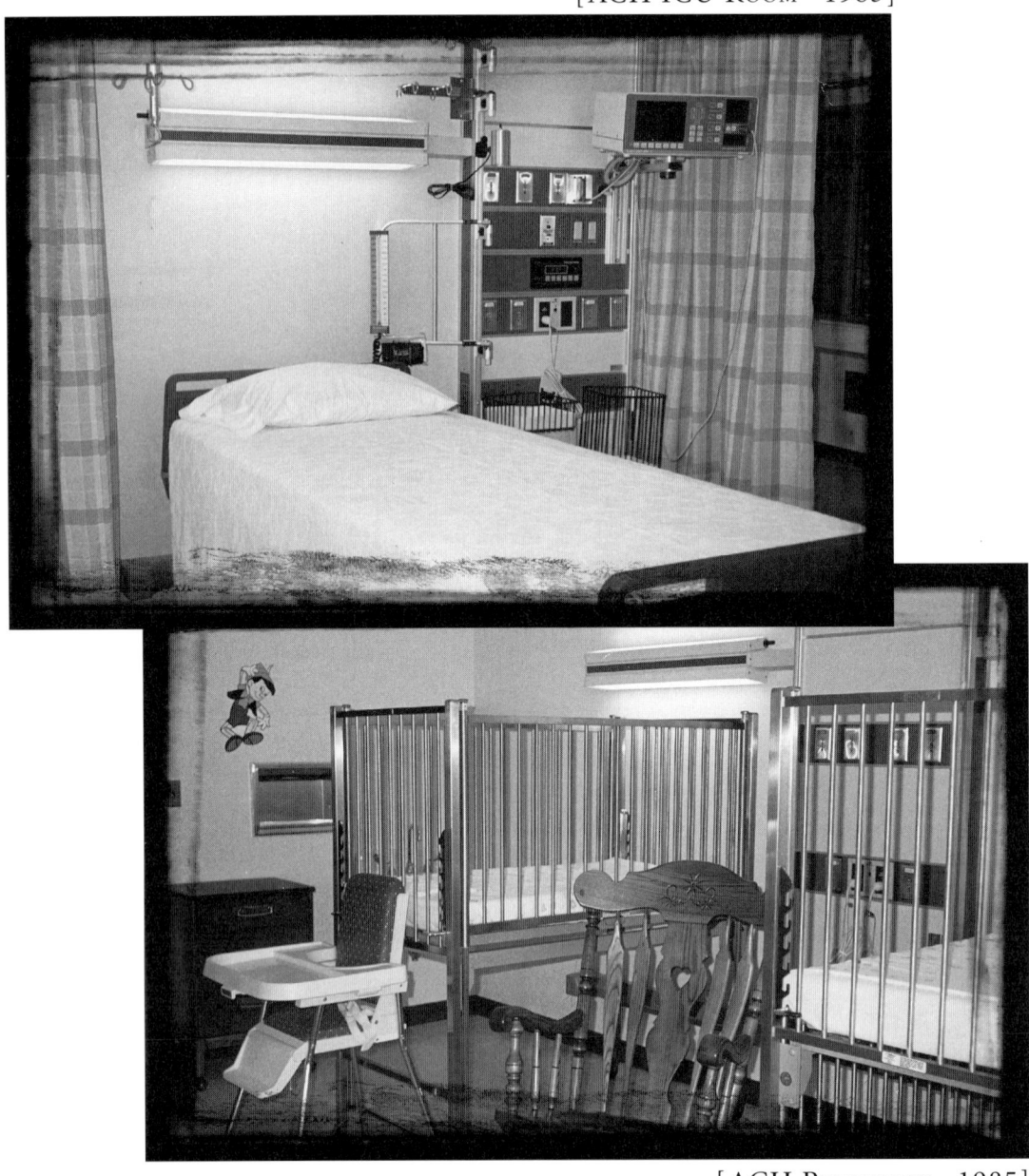

[ACH Pediatrics · 1985]

coming years: morale, communication, image, marketing, costs and financial issues, consistency with policies, reduction in administrative changes, and the need to be "first" in something. Financial priorities at this time were to control overtime, undertake a department by department manpower analysis, control supplies and increase materials management, and do a more thorough account analysis.[195]

1986 continued the exciting trends started

in 1985: better financial condition of the hospital and exciting new programs. 1986 also saw the hospital change its name for the third time in its history. The hospital, which had started as the Reformed Deaconess Home and Hospital and had spent the better part of the century as Alliance City Hospital, found itself wanting to emphasize its close relationship with the citizens of Alliance and thus, the hospital became Alliance Community Hospital. Along with this name change came an important change in corporate structure. Alliance Citizens' Health Association was formed at the same time as the name change to better emphasize the community nature of the hospital's mission. Indeed, according to the hospital's mission, it was to become a "community health care center."

The Citizens' Health Association had two specific roles: one was the hospital itself, another was the Alliance Community Foundation, a permanent development board that would remove the burden of fundraising from many of the medical professionals. According to the 1986 *Annual Report*, the Community Foundation's role was to "serve as an avenue to develop funds for new programs and services needed in our community." The Foundation is committed to the development of a philanthropic spirit through an ongoing program of fundraising activities to support the mission of the hospital. The fundraising activities include annual campaigns, memorial gifts, the annual Hospice Walk, Tree of Life ceremony, and other special campaigns.

1986 also saw many exciting new medical programs including the opening of the two new L-D-R (labor-delivery-recovery) suites in "The Birth Place", advanced eye surgery called radial keratotomy, and "Lifeline", a 24-hour-a-day "panic button" based emergency response service. Perhaps the most important project in 1986 was the training of all hospital staff in customer relations and a new administrative award for employee of the month. By the end of 1986 the hospital was also in good financial shape, reporting a total fund balance of $24,522,200.

Compared with the previous year, 1987 was a relatively quiet one. Major medical news involved the purchase of a General Electric CT 9000 scanner, which cost over $500,000, and the merger of Alliance Community Hospital with the Alliance Visiting Nurse Association, which would, according to the *Annual Report*, "make a more comprehensive array of services available to the patient and ... lead to a decrease in costs because of a cutback in hospital stays."

1987 was also the first full year of operation for the Community Cancer Center. The facility, which was the first of its type in Stark County, has over 9000 square feet of space for outpatient examination and treatment as well as room for inpatient care in both private and semiprivate rooms. The first director of the center was Dr. Angelo Demis, a specialist in hematology and oncology. The Cancer Center went a long way towards fulfilling CEO Melvin Pucci's claim that "the purpose of Alliance Community Hospital [is] compassionate care, quality care givers and a dedication to service and medical science."[196]

1988 was a year of growth for the hospital. Additions to the hospital's main physical plant featured the construction of the new front entrance, which included the enclosure of the canopy, new snack and gift shops, and a solarium. The hospital also expanded beyond its original boundaries with the completion of two projects: the Alliance Medical Services Building (currently the home of Immediately Medical Services) and the Marlington Family Practice Center in Marlboro Township.

Medical additions this year included the installation of EPIC [emergency patient instruction compiler] which helped serve as a clearinghouse for discharge instructions including a discussion of the diagnosis, natural course, potential complications, warning signs, and customary treatments of illnesses or injuries. The 1988 *Annual Report* also emphasizes the Outpatient Surgery Unit, which was designed to allow patients to have surgery and return home the same day, thus reducing cost and improving recovery time.

1989 saw the hospital end the eighties a strong, committed community institution. During this year they completed construction of the Medical Services Building on West State Street, which was to house Immediate Medical Services, Alliance Home Health Care, and Stark County Orthopedic Associates. The $1,000,000 "South Lawn Project" was also finished. This project included a new drive-up entrance from Arch Street and new offices for the Radiology Department.

The hospital ended the eighties a much different institution than it was when it began. Statistically, the hospital was down in nearly every category (admissions, births, laboratory procedures, &c.) but there were, in 1989, 53,504 outpatient clinic visits. In 1981 there were none. This indicates that Alliance Community Hospital was truly doing its job of providing total healthcare for the entire community, and if part of that meant not rushing to check people into the hospital and attempting to treat them on an outpatient basis, then so much the better, for the hospital and for the patient.

The nineties found the Alliance Community Hospital stronger than ever before. By the time the decade had ended, the hospital would see one more major renovation/addition and the signing of an agreement with Aultman Hospital that would position Alliance Community Hospital to become a major regional healthcare provider well into the next century.

Starting in 1994 the hospital undertook a fairly significant renovation of the emergency department "to better serve the increasing

[ACH CAFETERIA · 1985]

number of people who seek treatment there each year."[197] Other construction that started in 1994 included what the hospital was calling "the link" between the hospital and the community care center (the hospital's long-term care facility). This link would provide "easier access to hospital services for center residents." An addition was completed to the aforementioned care center and improvements were made to the loading docks and storage areas. 1994 also saw the opening of a remodeled ado-

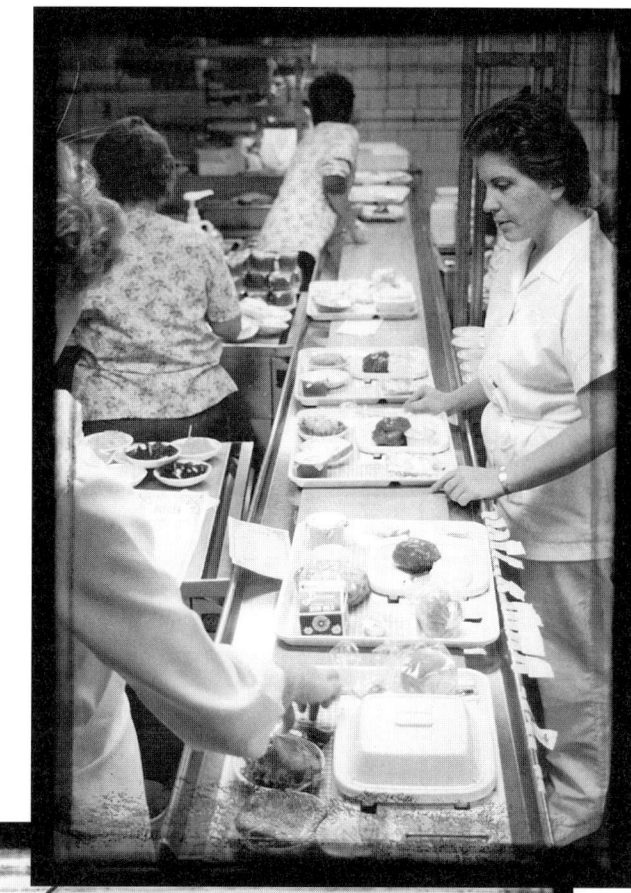

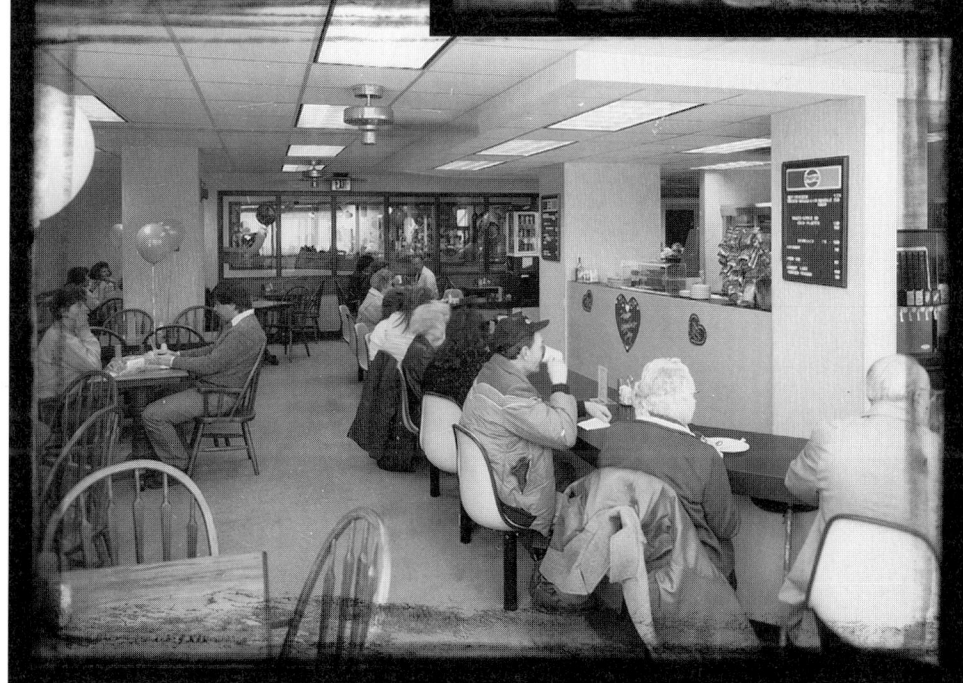

[ACH SNACK SHOP · 1985]

lescent and pediatric care unit that featured "a colorful carousel theme and . . . large playroom in sight of the nurse's station."

1994 also saw the departure of CEO Melvin Pucci, who had been with the hospital for nine years. Pucci was replaced by James Bingham, who came to Alliance from Louisiana.

1995 saw a number of excellent accomplishments: "Two million dollars in federal grants, national recognition of our rehabilitation department, the installation of several pieces of new equipment and progress toward a new emergency room" were just some of the achievements of Mr. Bingham's first year.[198] The grants, acquired with the help of Representative Ralph Regula and Senator John Glenn, were for improvements in community wellness and the continued additions to the Community Care Center.

1995 also saw the approval by the City Planning Commission of the 10,000 square foot expansion of the emergency room facilities. Included in the plans were eight general examining rooms including a pediatric room and a "fast track" area to handle non-urgent medical problems. The total estimated cost of the expansion was set at $3,000,000. Most of the addition would be paid for out of hospital operating funds, and a combination of bonds and donations, including an especially large gift from the Timken Foundation; over $500,000 came from monies raised by the Auxiliary and the Alliance Community Hospital Foundation.[199]

1996 saw several new programs and services and the breaking of ground on the new Emergency facilities (set to open in June 1997). According to the *Annual Report*, new programs this year included the new Wellness Department and the *Wellness Challenge*—a relationship between the hospital and local companies that created an incentive-based program to reduce company healthcare costs. The first companies to be included in this program were Alliance Community Hospital, Alliance Midwest Tubular Products, and Alliance Machine.

Other new programs in 1996 included the Mother/Baby program, inpatient Dialysis Services, Water Therapy, and the creation of a web page for the hospital.

1997 was the most significant year in the nineties for a number of reasons. The opening of the new emergency facilities in June gave the hospital a modern trauma center able to deal with a variety of problems. The hiring of new CEO Stan Jonas saw the addition of stability to an office that had seen three CEOs in three years.

The Emergency Center was an impressive building. According to the hospital's own records, the facility was built "with the flexibility to respond to the ever-changing needs of the community and the health care industry."[200] According to Jonas, the hospital was dedicating itself to "patient and customer service," and would devote much of the energy of the hospital to "paying attention to details, caring, delighting, providing comfort and compassion." The hospital also moved towards the future by starting a formal credentialing process for midwives, certified nurse anesthetists, and physicians' assistants. 1997 also saw the creation of the full-time position of chaplain, which is supported by the hospital auxiliary.

A CENTURY OF CARING

The Future

The Future

In 1900, the Reformed Deaconess Home and Hospital was formed. With it came the original mission "... to care for the sick, whether physically or spiritually, and to engage in such other forms of charitable and benevolent work which may commend themselves to the association." As Alliance Community Hospital begins its second century of service to the people of Alliance, it builds upon these principles with the following present-day Mission and Vision Statements:

> Alliance Community Hospital exists to provide quality healthcare and services with absolute caring from the heart.
>
> The Vision of Alliance Community Hospital is to become the premier community hospital in the State of Ohio.

At the beginning of its second century, the Hospital has more than 900 colleagues, more than 150 volunteers, over 80 active physicians on staff, and more than 250 beds. In the year 2000 there were 5,318 inpatient admissions, 23,133 emergency room visits, 86,700 outpatient services performed, 50,310 Visiting Nurse and Hospice visits, and 15,549 visits to Immediate Medical Services, the urgent care facility on West State Street.

In September 1999 the Hospital signed a joint venture agreement with Aultman Hospital of Canton, Ohio, gaining access to capital funding based on a shared vision of maintaining a strong, locally owned and governed, not-for-profit Community Hospital. This agreement, along with Alliance's strong financial performance over the last five years, will allow ACH to move ahead with its replacement hospital and medical campus. The new facilities (called the Healthcare Campus) will provide the citizens of the Alliance Area with a "modern, attractive, and customer-friendly hospital; extended care facility (ECF); and administrative and medical office building."

Key aspects of the design of the facilities are based on customer feedback and focus groups conducted throughout 2001 and 2002. Those aspects include a customer-friendly design with the patients and their families as the core concern; vast majority of rooms will be private (one patient); smaller nursing units called PODS; and more centralized outpatient services.

The expansion included the purchase of several homes and buildings to the south and west of the hospital, as well as the land under what is currently State Street Middle School and the Family Medical Arts Building. Without these additional properties, the new campus could not have been built on the present site.

Although the process of acquiring the properties was not easy for those being asked to leave homes, the hospital acted in a manner that most would consider a good neighbor. At great expense, one homeowner's house was moved across the street for the benefit of the son, and another building was donated to Habitat for Humanity. According to residents Beth and Randy Miles, "The hospital and its representatives acted very fairly. We are using the money from the sale of our home to build a larger home in (a) less commercial area."[202]

The year 1999 also saw ACH joining the Northeast Ohio Health Network. This is a group of hospitals, including Dunlap Memorial Hospital in Orrville, Joel Pomerene Hospital in Millersburg, and Union Hospital in Dover, that are dedicated to "providing people with preventative health information and services" that will increase their quality of life.[203]

Several new programs, services, or departments were started or refurbished in 1999. These included a new Cardiac Rehabilitation department, the addition of a Lactation Consultant, a Voice-Activated Operating Room System, and Sleep Lab studies.

The hospital entered its 100th year of service to the community of Alliance as a vital center of healthcare for everyone. The hospital continued to add new services, including the Senior Care Gero-Psychiatry unit (specifically designed to "address the emotional and medical needs of older adults so that they may maintain a satisfying quality of life");[204] a Mobile Health Unit charged with providing "wellness and prevention programming for the communities and services of Alliance Community Hospital, Dunlap Memorial Hospital, Joel Pomerene Hospital, and Union Hospital (Northeast Ohio Health Network), and the Access Alliance project, which provided "individuals who are physically challenged and their families educational and practical experiences which enable them to actively participate in community interests."

The new hospital campus project made great strides forward in 2000; the first visible sign of the development was the building of a new parking lot and heliport on the west side of the hospital. The Burt Hill Kosar Rittelman Associates Healthcare Design Group was chosen to provide architectural and engineering services for the new campus.

Groundbreaking for the new campus officially began on April 24, 2002 for the Administrative and Medical Office Building.

The year 2000 also saw the relocation of the Good Samaritan Clinic to the Alliance Neighborhood Center. The building, the former St. Joseph School, was donated by the Hospital to become the Alliance Neighborhood Center. Many of the hospital's staff, including physicians, nurses, and technicians, work in the clinic on a volunteer basis or serve on the Board of Trustees. The hospital also initiated a fundraising golf event—The Charity Care Classic—that benefits the clinic. The Good Samaritan Clinic continues to be a real help to those citizens of Alliance who are without any healthcare.

The year 2000 saw the hospital looking at itself and taking stock of where it had been and where it hoped to go. Several events celebrating the hospital's Centennial were planned, and a Centennial Plaza was created in front of the main entrance. By the end of 2000, more than $90,000 had been donated or earmarked for this fund. This amount was just a small part of the over $1,000,000 disbursed from the Foundation to assist the hospital since 1990.

According to Hospital CEO Stan Jonas, the last five years (1997-2001) have been as important a time in the hospital's history as any in the previous 100. "The hospital has been made ready," Jonas commented in an interview, "to face the increasingly challenging mission of continuing our tradition of absolute caring from the heart."[205] In remarks made at a ceremony for the end of the Centennial fund drive, Jonas elaborated saying that the hospital is "an army of doctors, nurses, and skilled health care professionals who always intend to be at the heart of the community." Jonas's goals for the future include continuing to grow the hospital at an acceptable rate while serving the communities' needs, and to "continue to use the best people and the best processes to achieve the best service" for all citizens of Alliance and the surrounding area.[206] Jonas also commented on the strong community leadership from the voluntary Boards of Trustees noting that they have been "the stability and foundation for keeping our hospital locally owned and governed. They have provided wonderful support whenever called upon by our administrative and medical staff leadership, and they have always been there when needed."

In May 2001, the hospital showed that they were indeed ready to care for all of the citizens of Alliance. During Memorial Day weekend, two students at West Branch High School, Jonathan Stauffer and Kelly Coblentz, died within 24 hours of each other from the same strain of bacterial meningitis. According to the *Alliance Review*, the Emergency Room at ACH was "flooded" with concerned parents and students, many of whom "waited in the lobbies and outside the sliding glass doors of the hospital . . . armed with questions and concerns about the infection and seeking preventative medication".[207] In response to the emergency conditions, the hospital set up a triage area in the outpatient department and distributed literature about the disease, including what kinds of antibiotics were being given, who was at risk for catching the disease, and what steps should be taken should someone feel they have symptoms. While there was some grumbling by local citizens about two- or three-hour waits, for the most part people were happy with the way the hospital handled the initial outbreak. When a third student, Christin VanCamp of Marlington High School, was diagnosed with a similar infection, the hospital literally threw open its doors and distributed over 29,000 doses of antibiotics to nearly every citizen of Alliance and the surrounding areas. Starting at 9:00 AM on Saturday, 2 June, the hospital distributed antibiotics and had medical staff on call for anyone who came by. There was no discussion of cost, or insurance, or liability—the hospital simply, calmly, and professionally fulfilled its obligation to the city of Alliance.[208]

On Saturday night, from around 6:00 PM until midnight, my wife and I waited in line with others for antibiotics. It was a truly remarkable situation. There was no panic or anger—everyone was there together, rich or poor, old or young. People were making coffee runs and sharing umbrellas and trading pens and pencils and exchanging books and magazines. When a helicopter landed on Saturday night with a new supply of antibiotics, a large cheer went up from the exhausted crowd. And many people volunteered. Two young people I met while waiting in line told me that they had come by around 10:00 that morning to get their antibiotics and had ended up staying to help pass out information sheets and pencils. CEO Stan Jonas told me in an interview that he was in the lobby around midnight helping to call out names and helping to keep up the spirits of a severely overworked medical staff and hospital personnel. An editorial in the *Alliance Review* on the Monday following the distribution summed it all up nicely: "Those who were gathered at the Alliance Community Hospital were met with medical kindness and expertise. The organized way in which our hospital enacted its disaster plan should give us all a sense of security".[209] Indeed, it does. The hospital lived up to its mission that day. Dr. Tressel and Reverend Kilmer just might be proud of what the hospital was able to accomplish.

The Alliance Community Hospital family looks forward to serving the community for the next 100 years.

A CENTURY OF CARING

Photo Gallery

CARING FOR OUR COMMUNITY

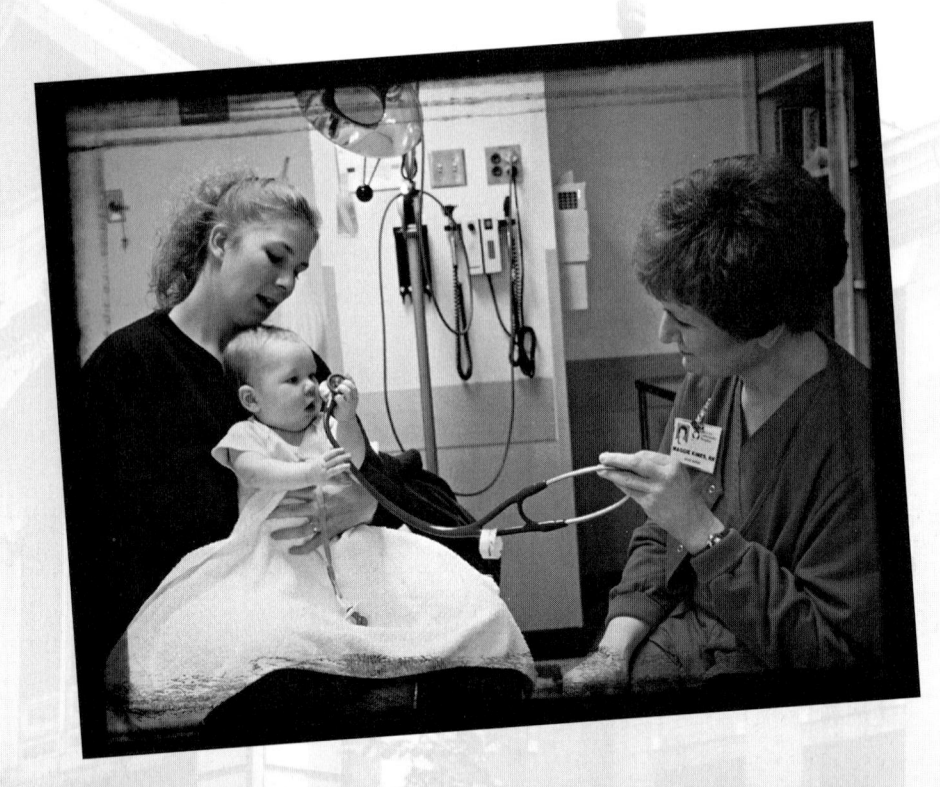

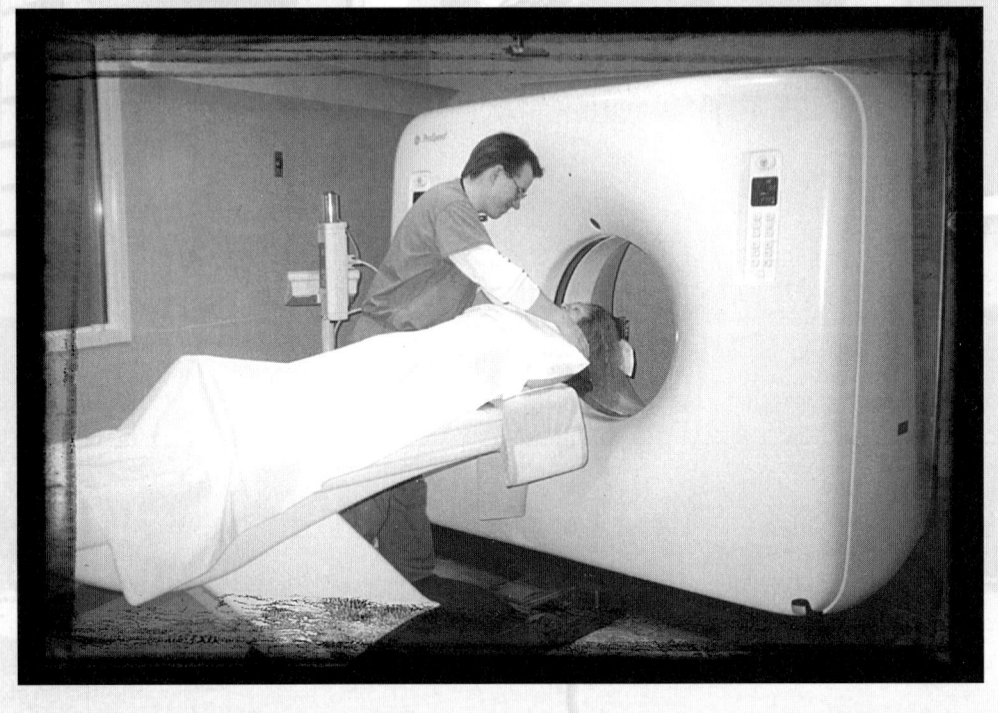

102 · *Photo Gallery* A CENTURY OF CARING

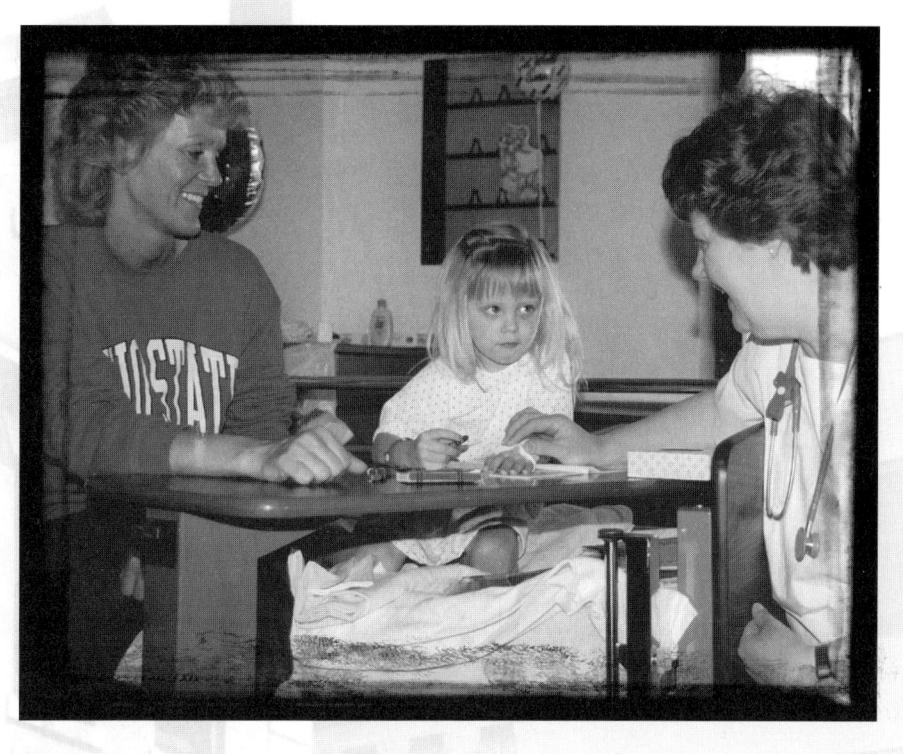

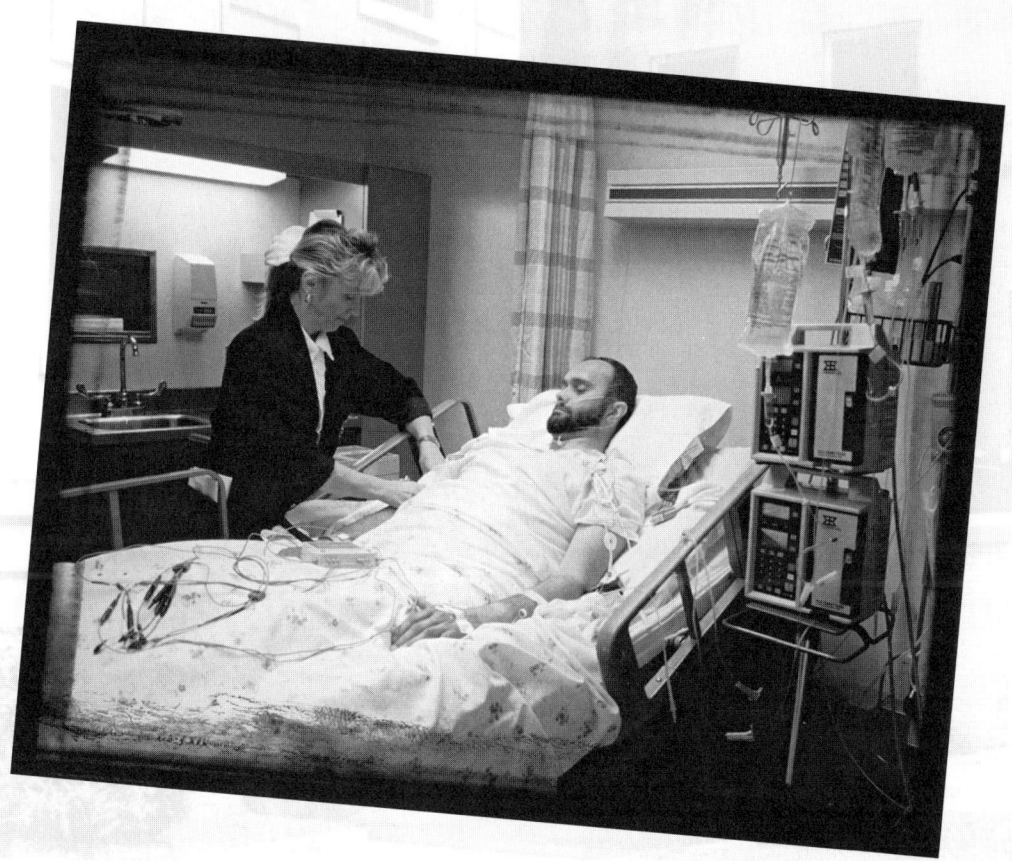

A CENTURY OF CARING *Photo Gallery* · 103

CARING FOR OUR COMMUNITY

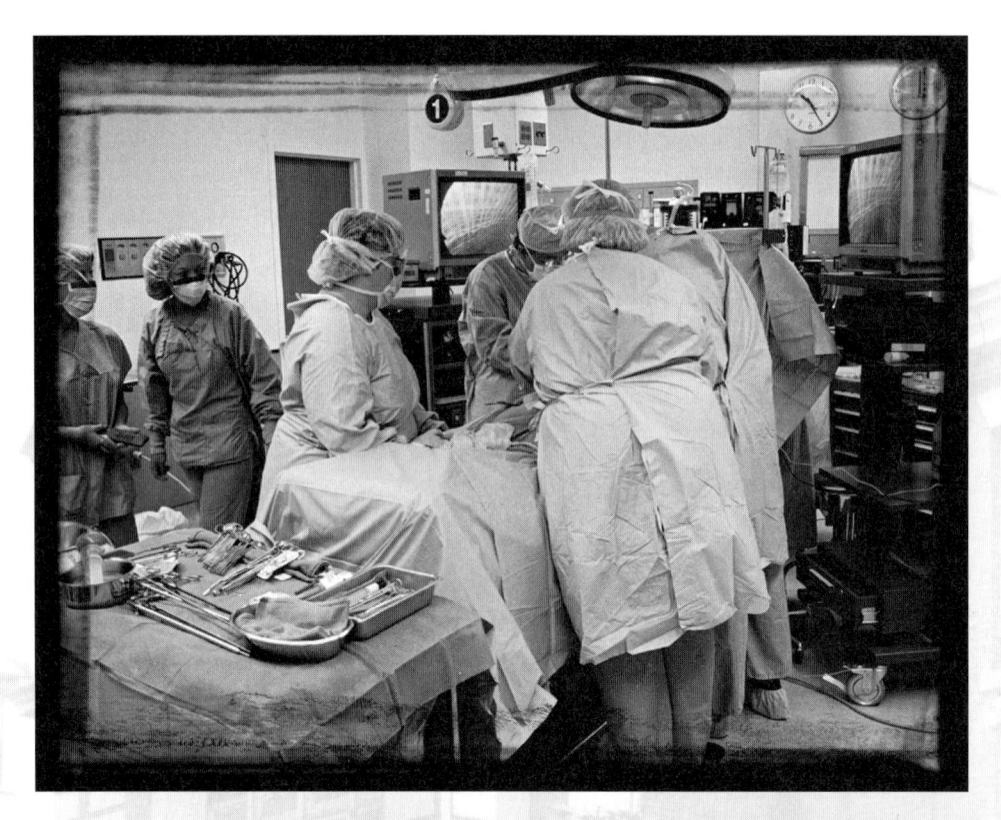

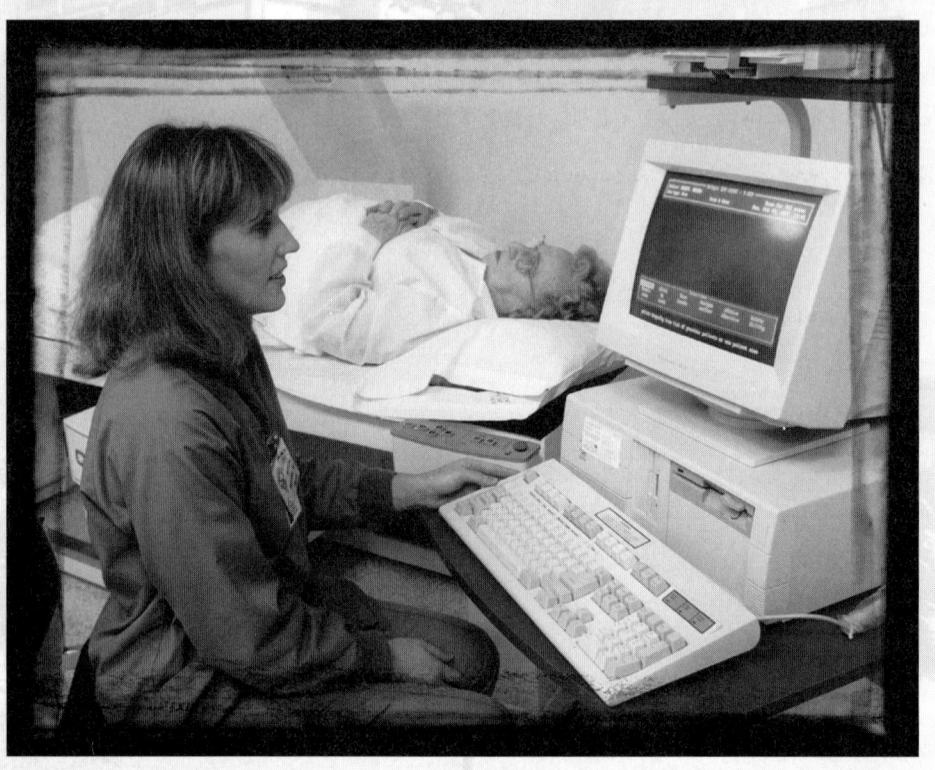

104 · *Photo Gallery*   A CENTURY OF CARING

CARING FOR OUR COMMUNITY

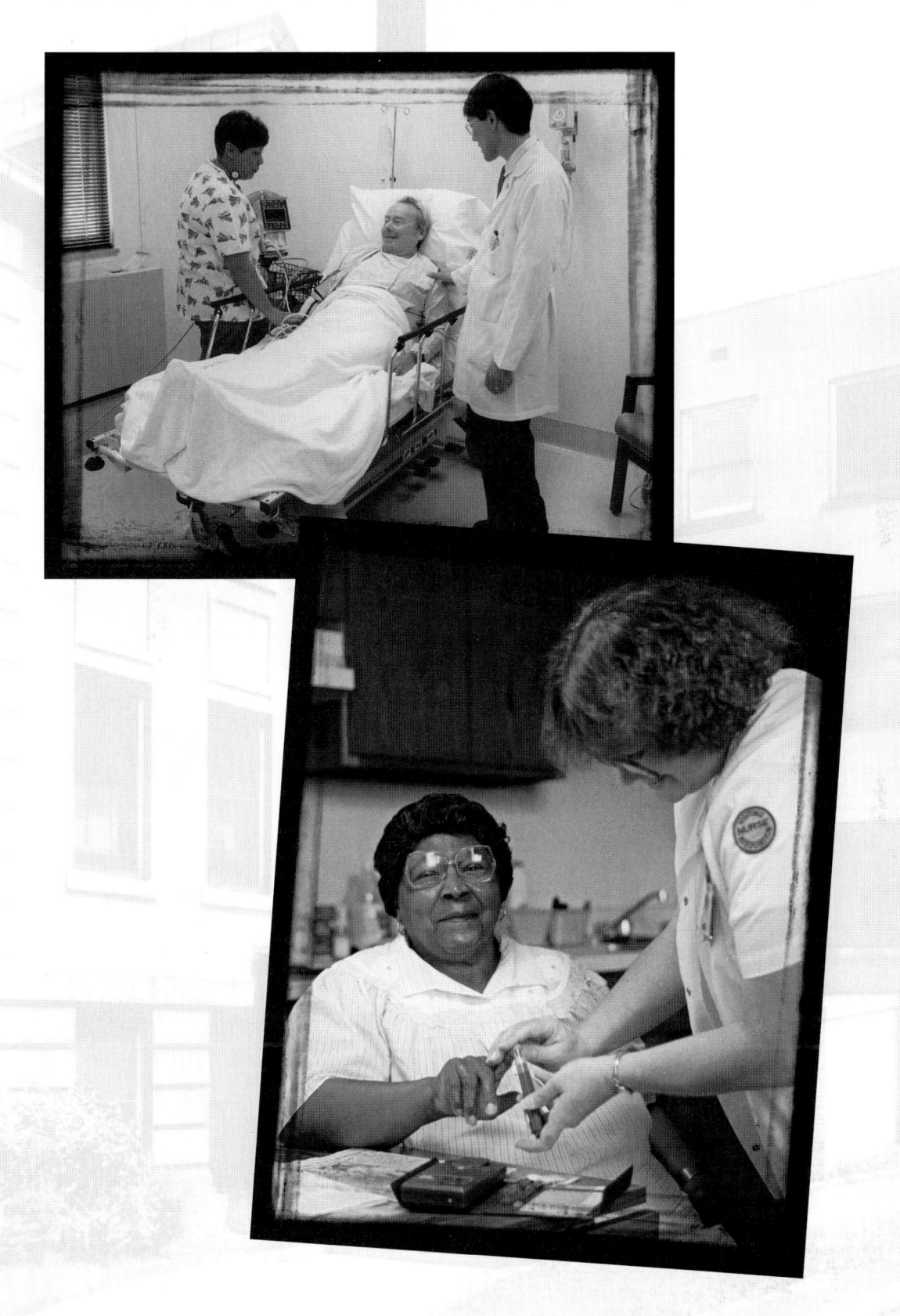

A CENTURY OF CARING *Photo Gallery* · 105

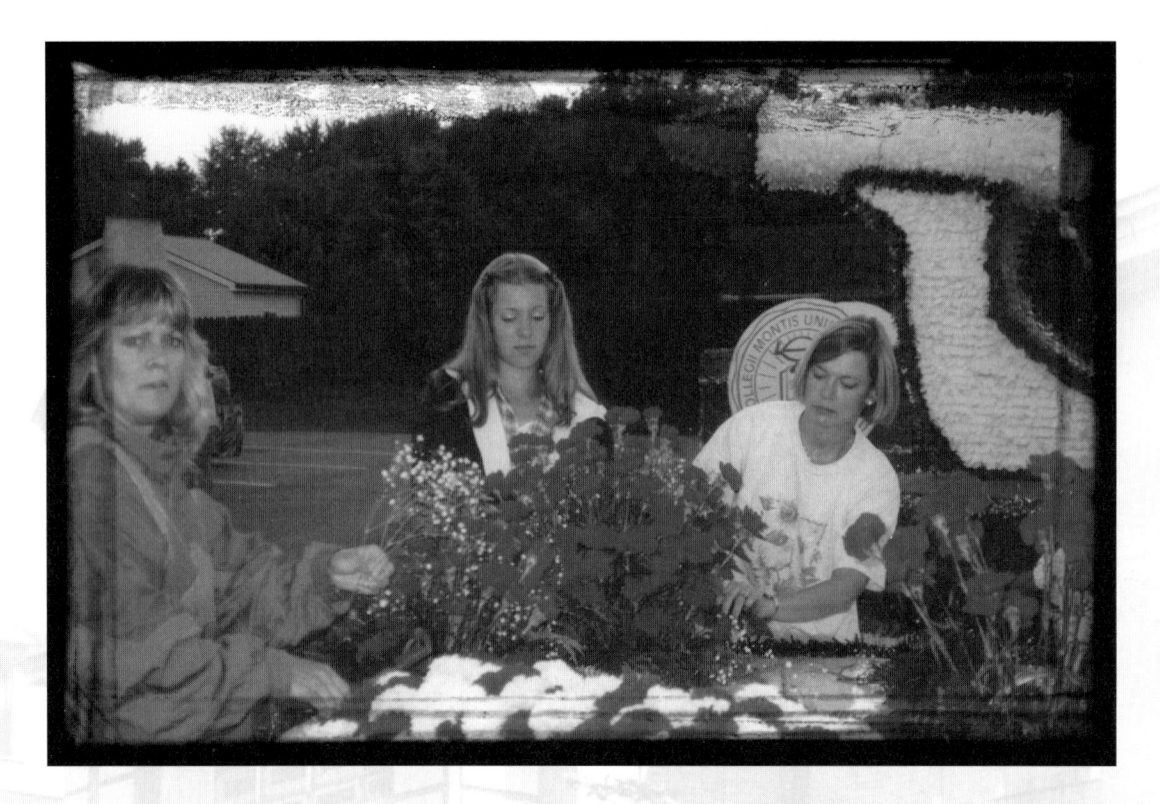

CARNATION DAYS

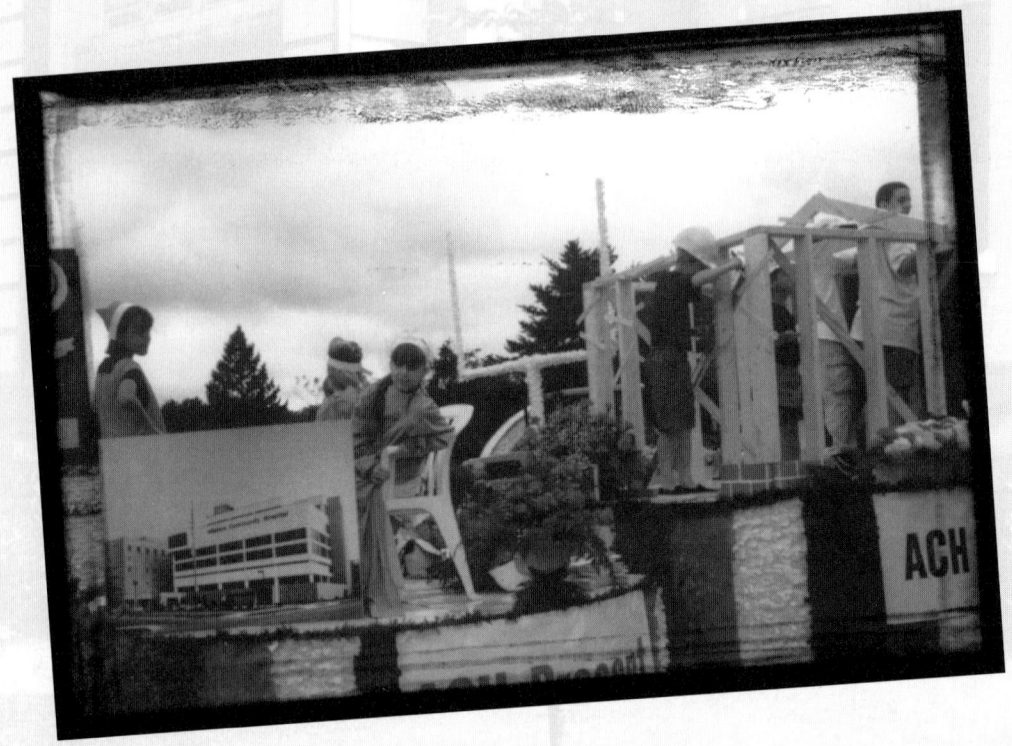

106 · *Photo Gallery*　A CENTURY OF CARING

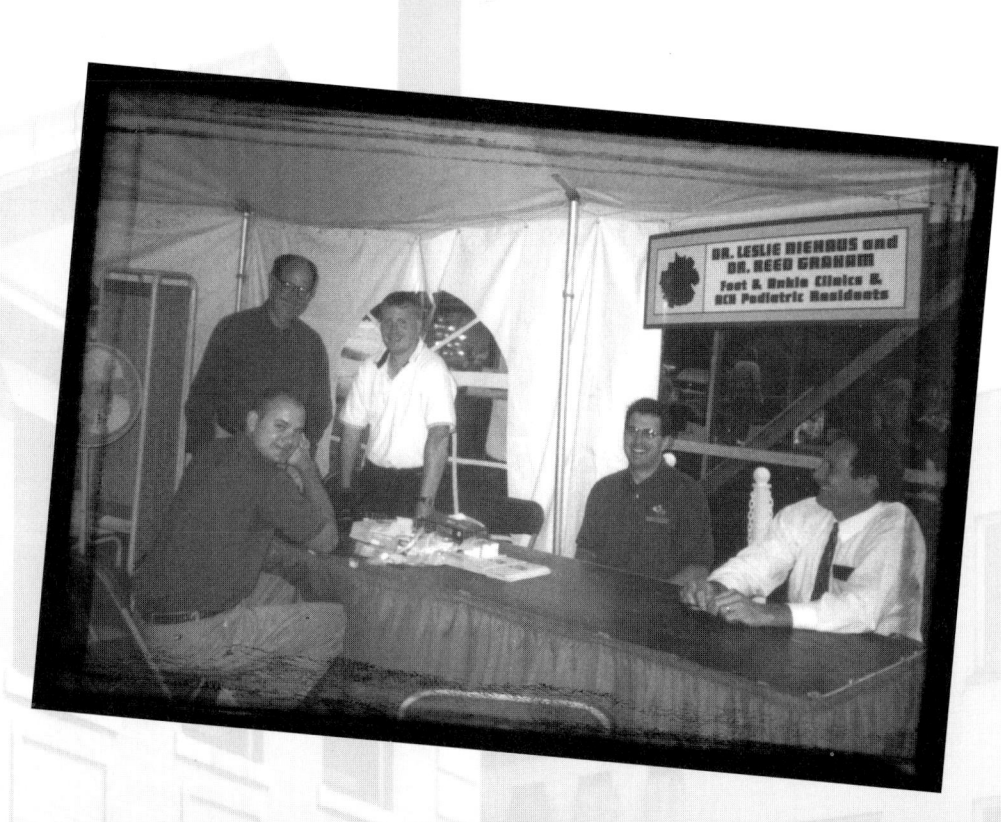

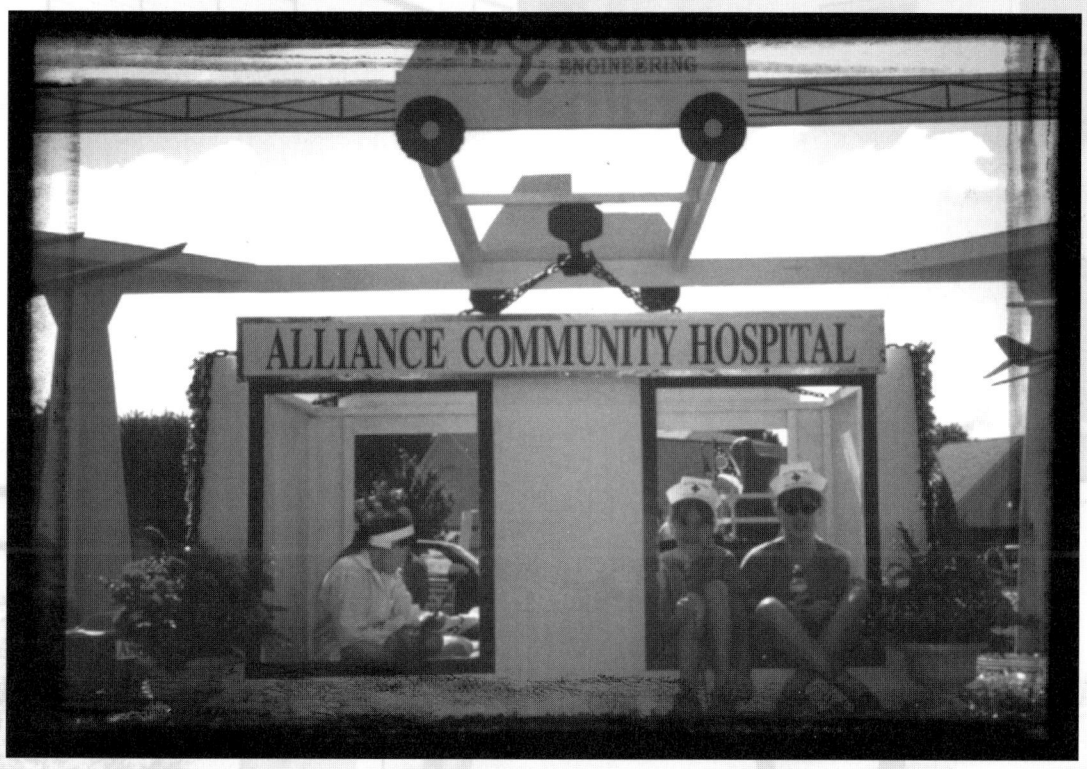

A CENTURY OF CARING   *Photo Gallery* · 107

CARNATION DAYS

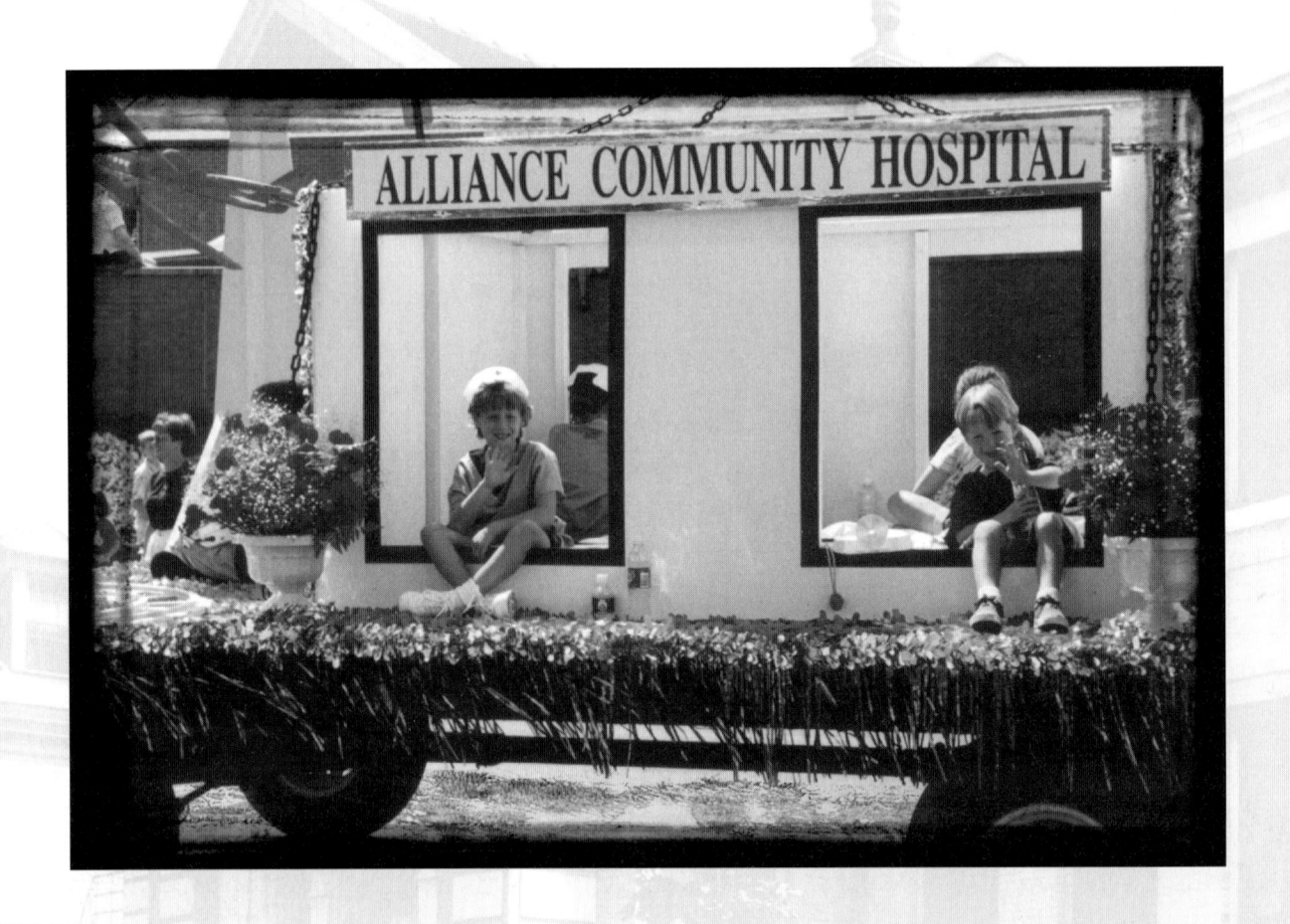

108 · *Photo Gallery*   A CENTURY OF CARING

CENTER FOR REHABILITATION
ACTIVITIES

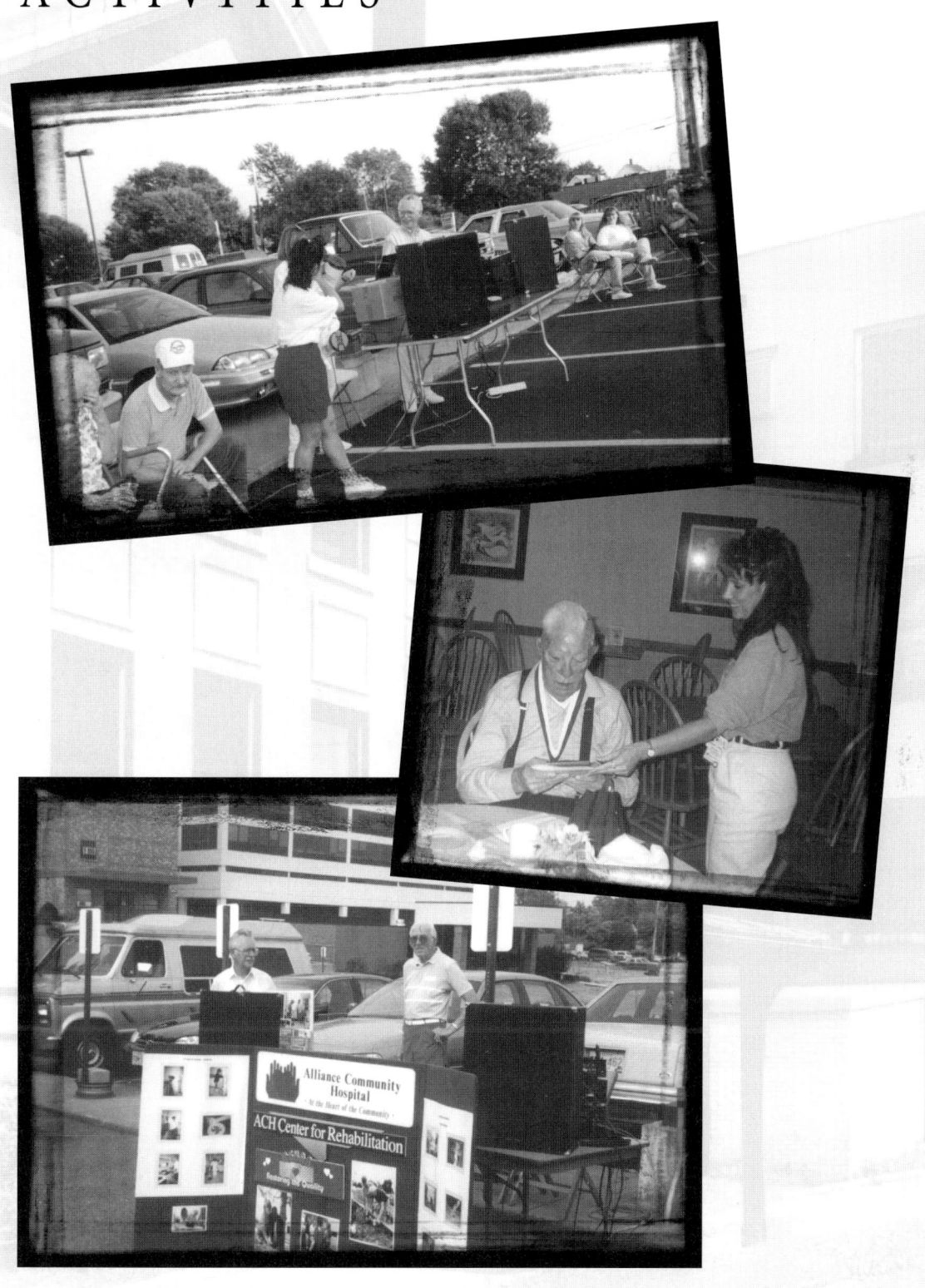

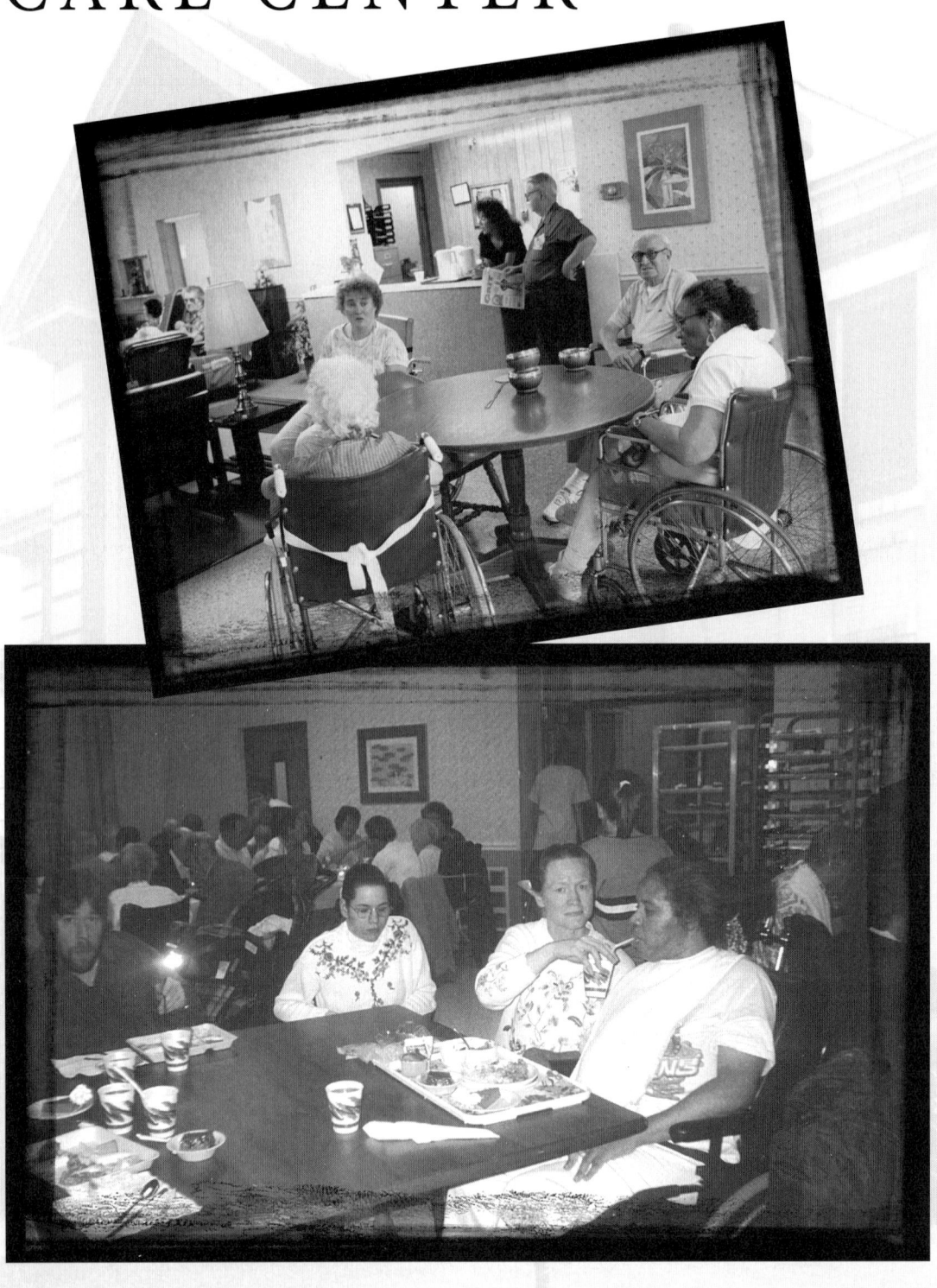

COMMUNITY CARE CENTER

110 · *Photo Gallery* A CENTURY OF CARING

COMMUNITY CARE CENTER

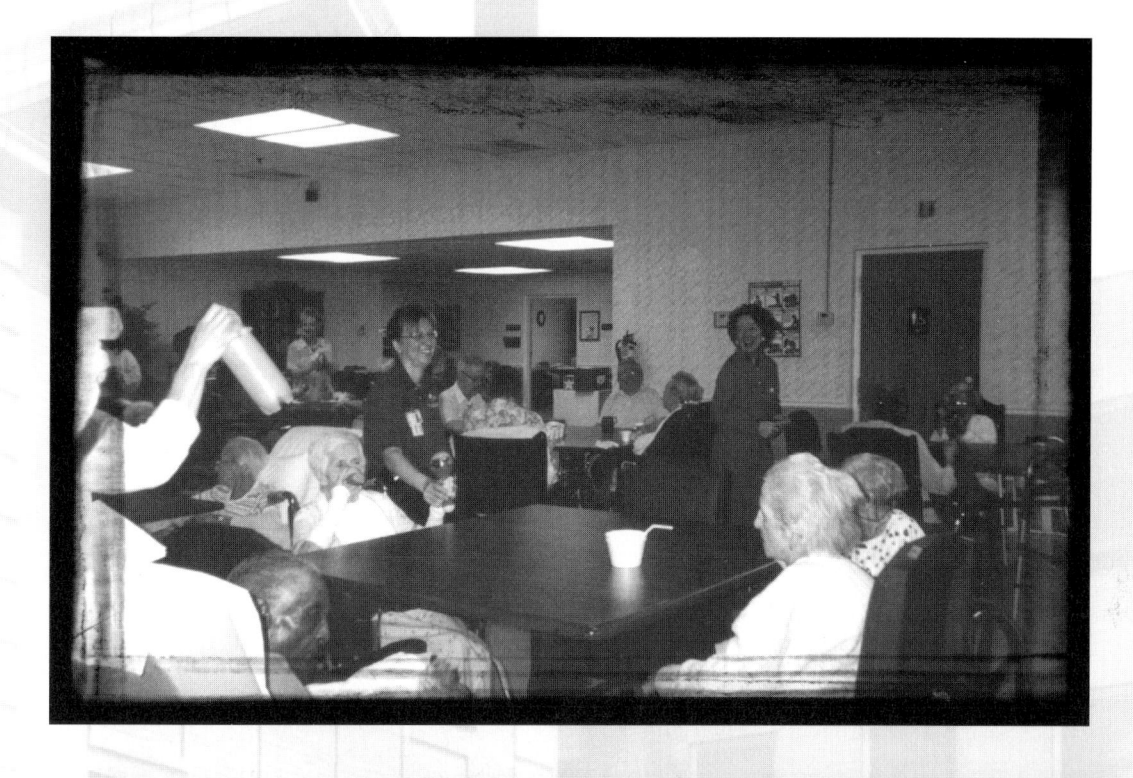

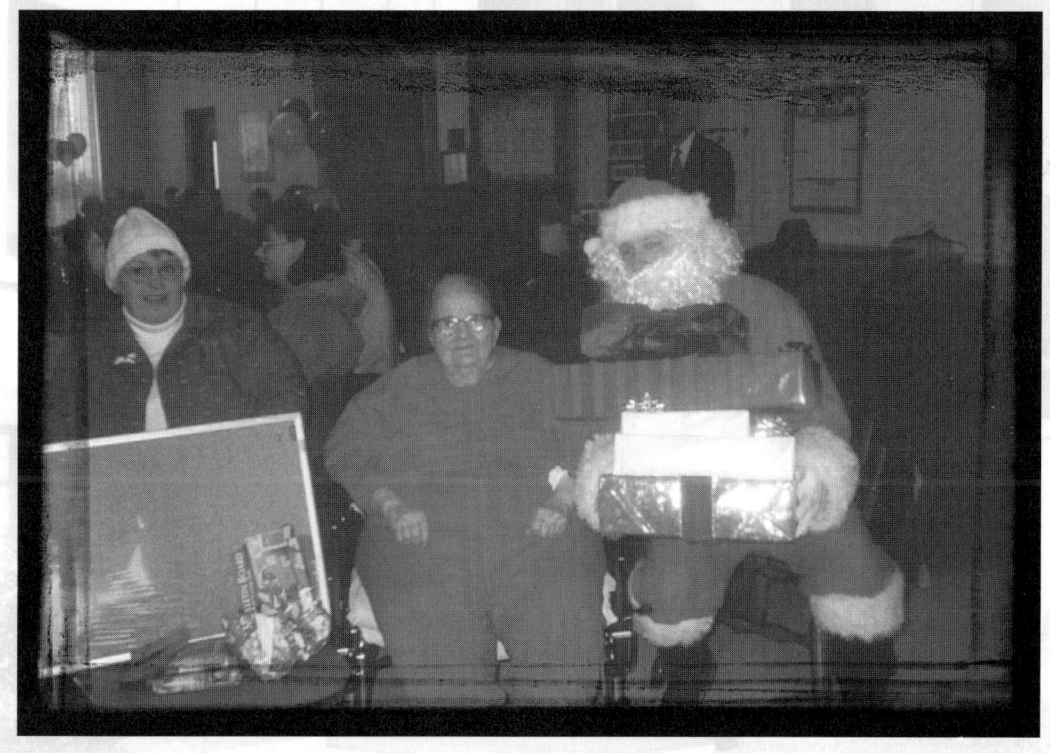

A CENTURY OF CARING · *Photo Gallery* · 111

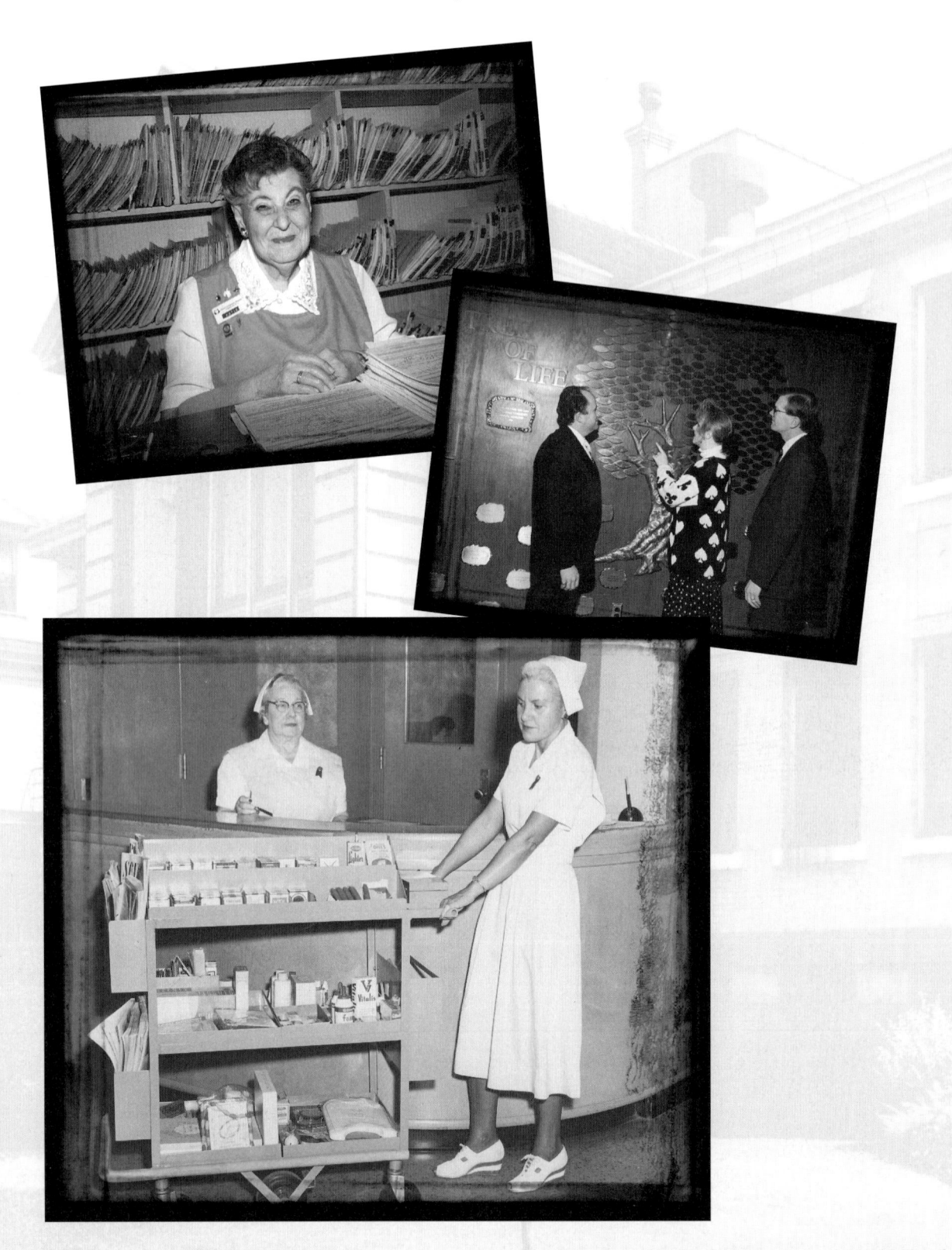

FOUNDATION/VOLUNTEERS

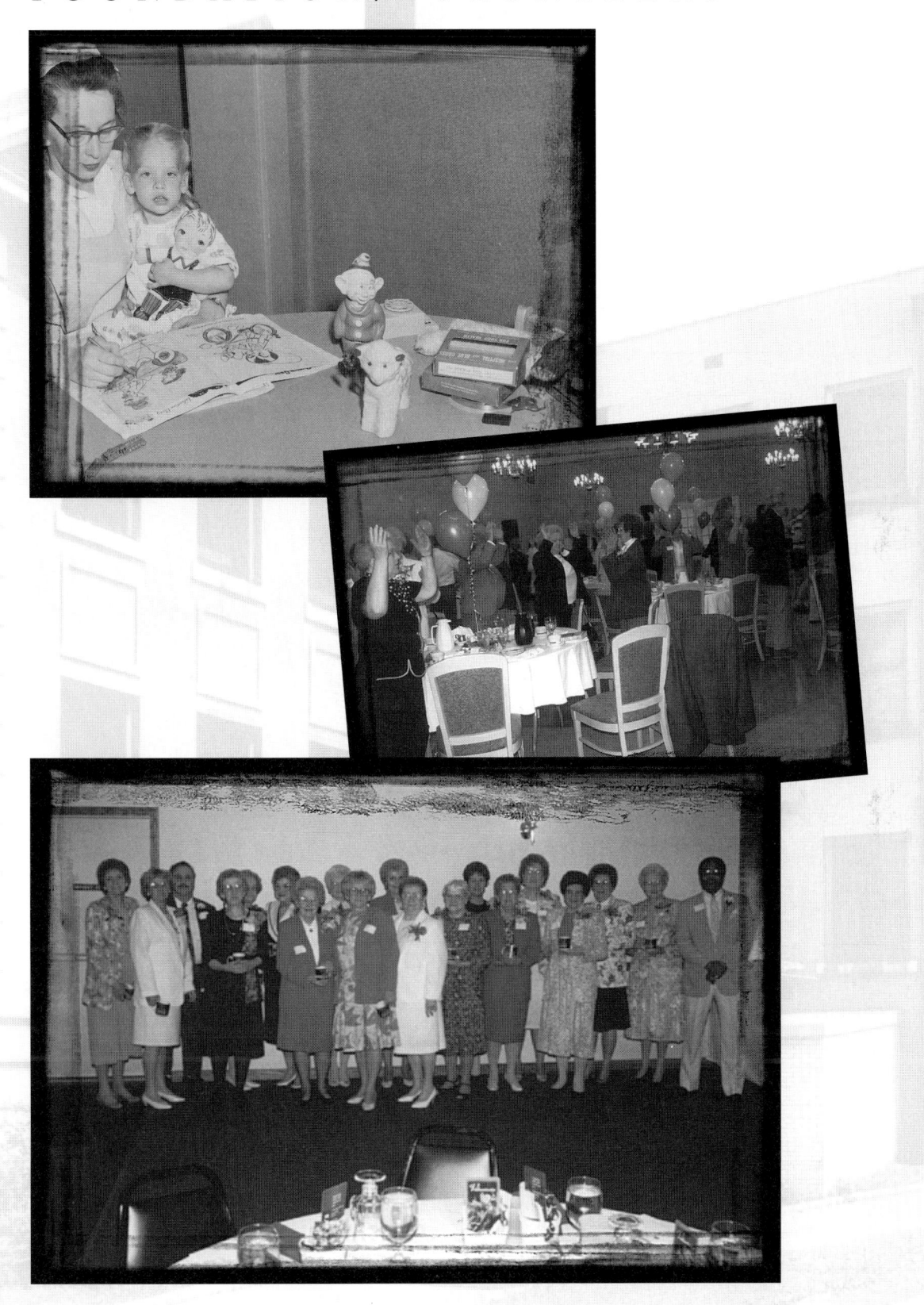

FOUNDATION/VOLUNTEERS

A CENTURY OF CARING *Photo Gallery* · 113

FOUNDATION/VOLUNTEERS

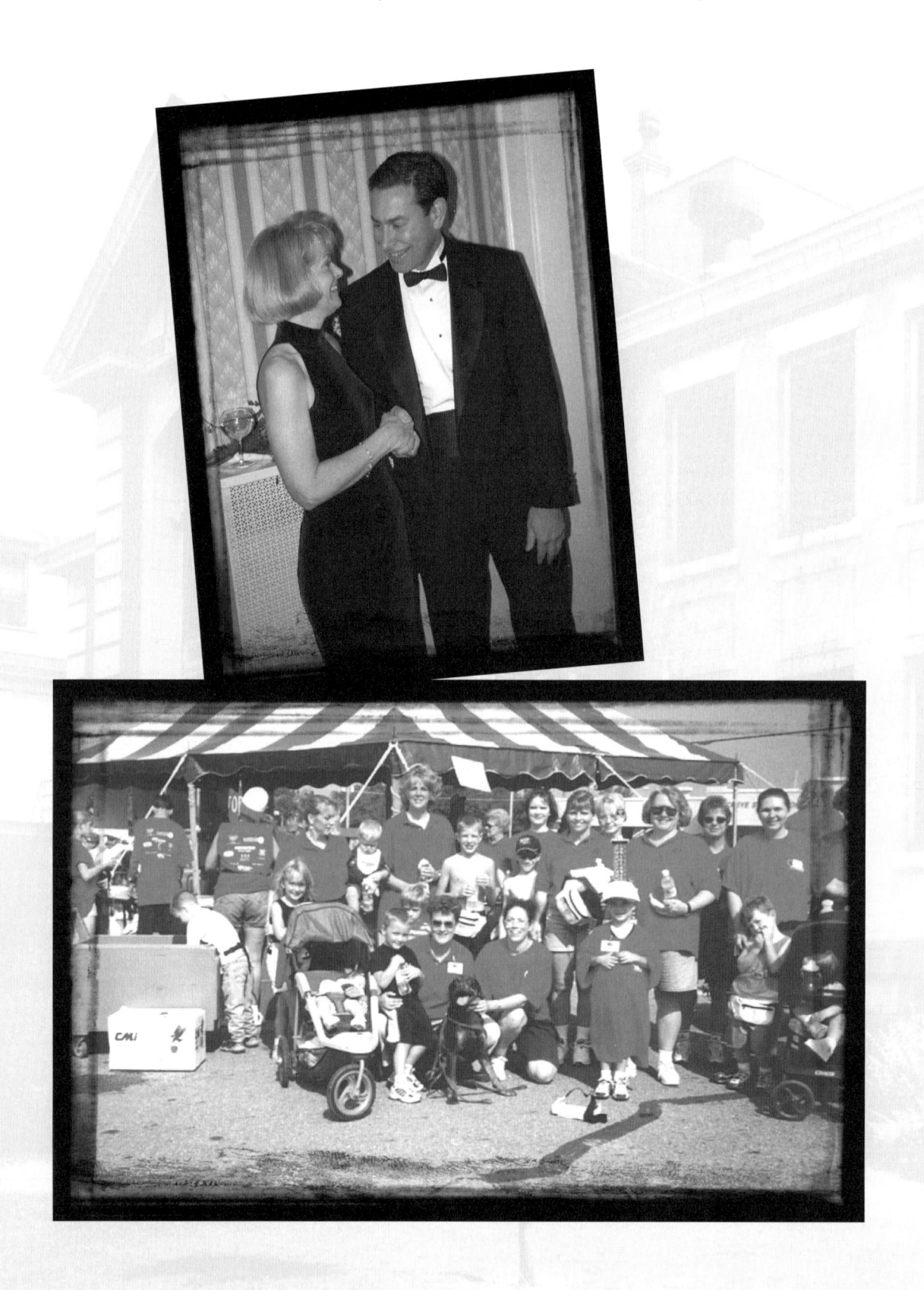

114 · *Photo Gallery* A CENTURY OF CARING

COMMUNITY CHALLENGE

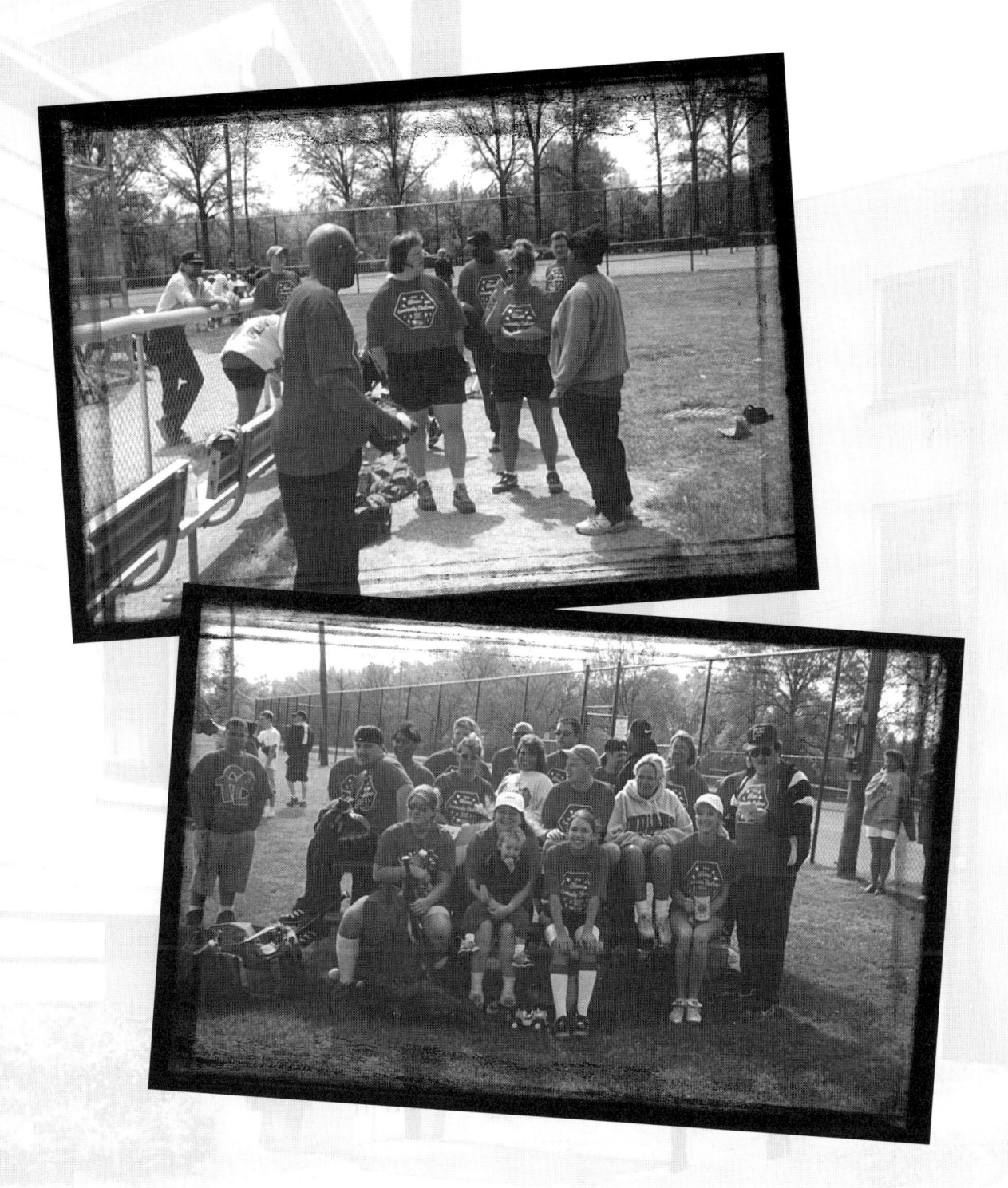

A CENTURY OF CARING *Photo Gallery* · 115

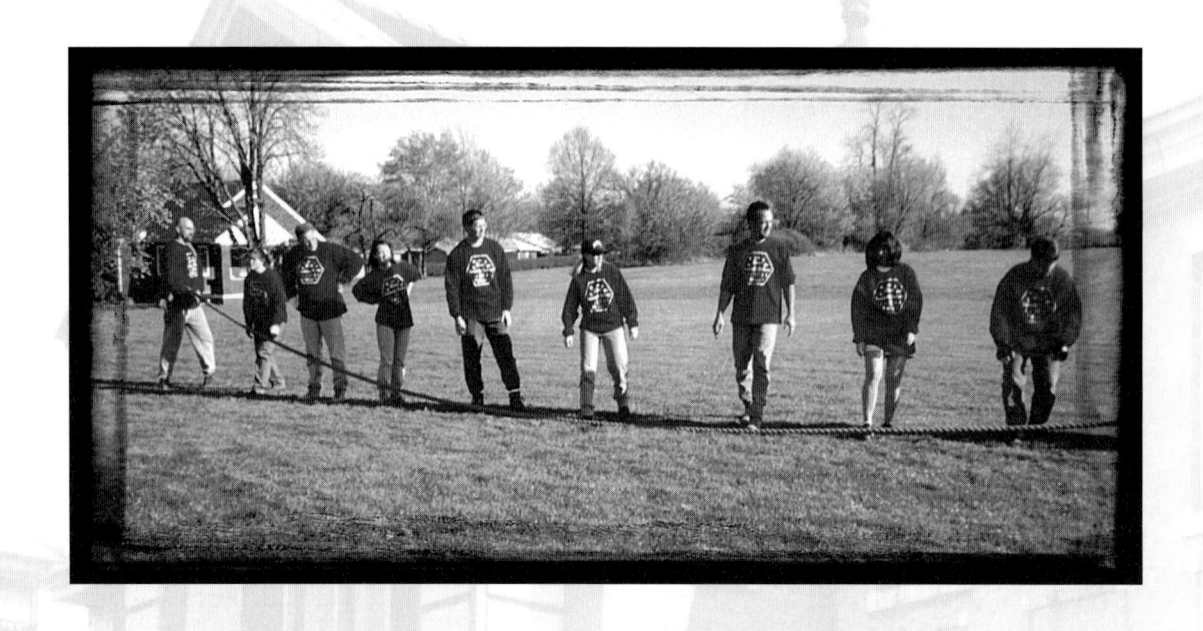

COMMUNITY CHALLENGE

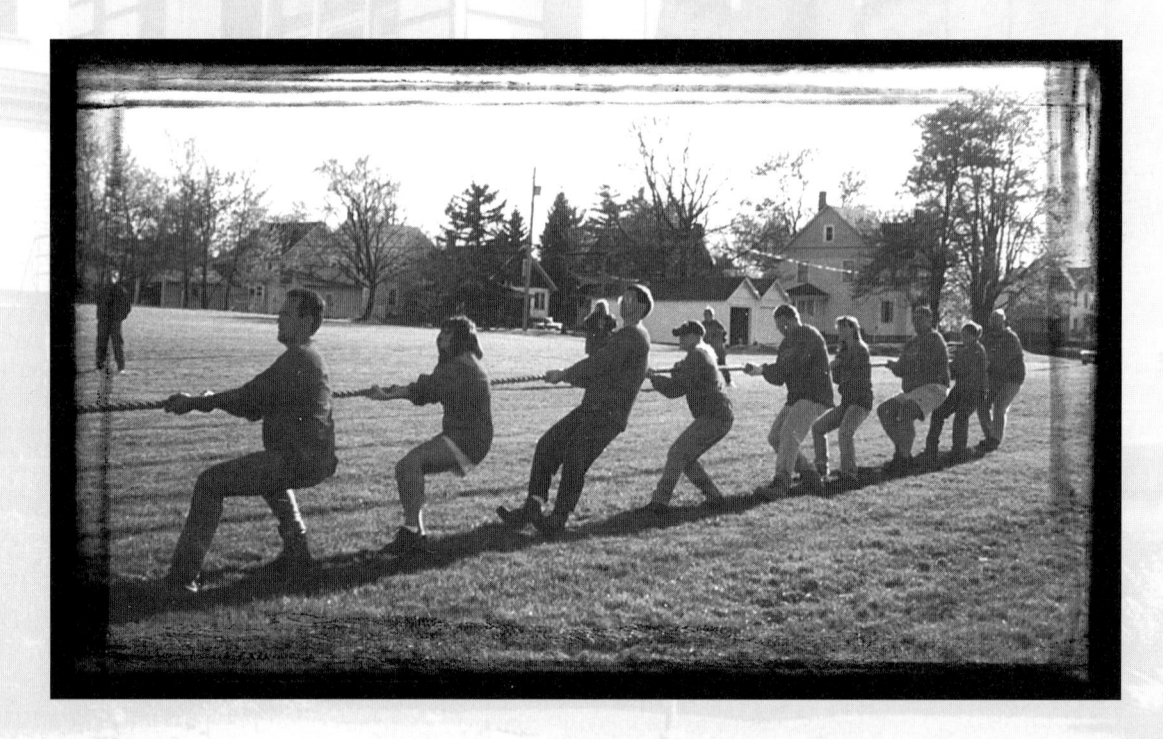

116 · *Photo Gallery*   A CENTURY OF CARING

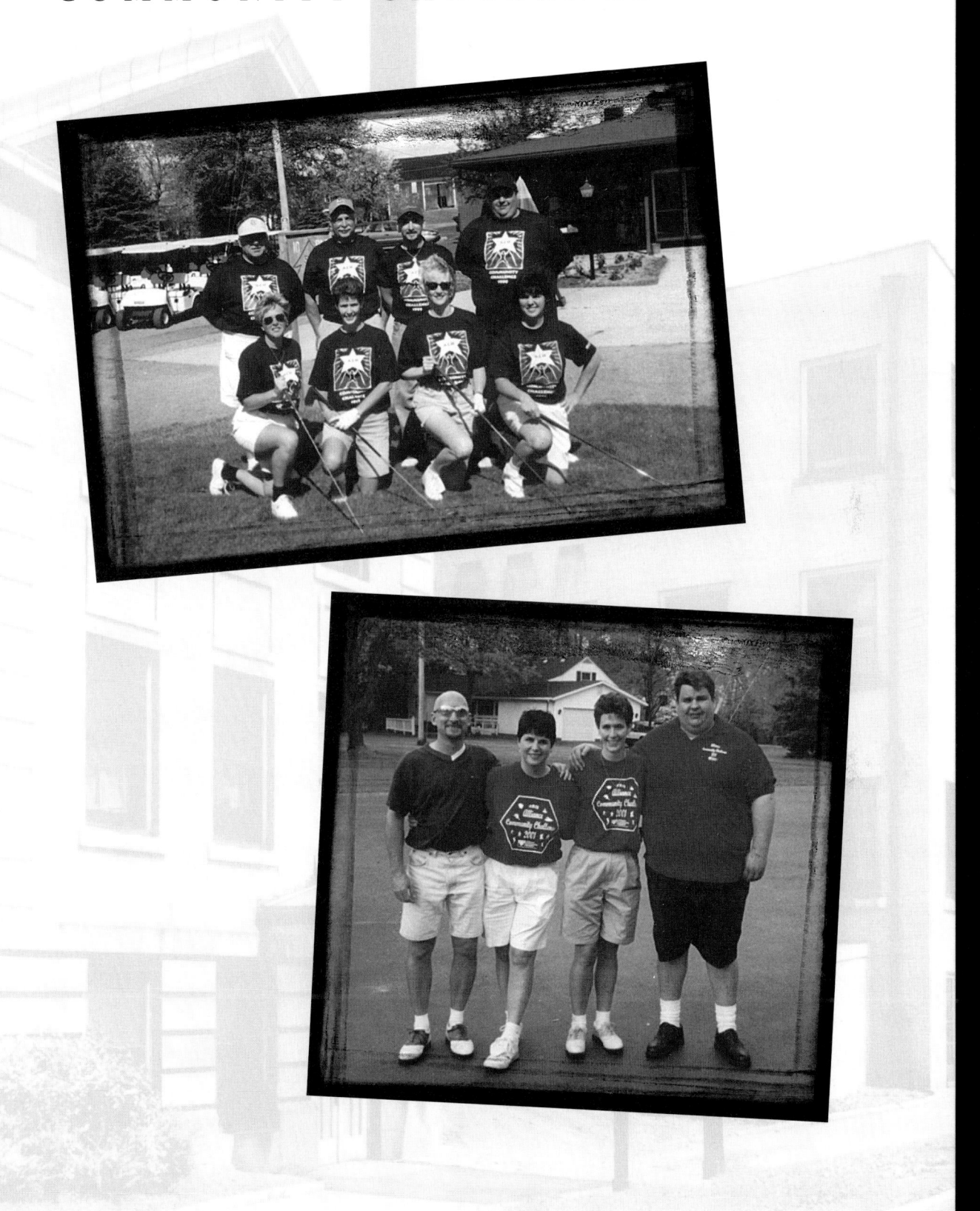

COMMUNITY CHALLENGE

A CENTURY OF CARING   *Photo Gallery* · 117

COMMUNITY CHALLENGE

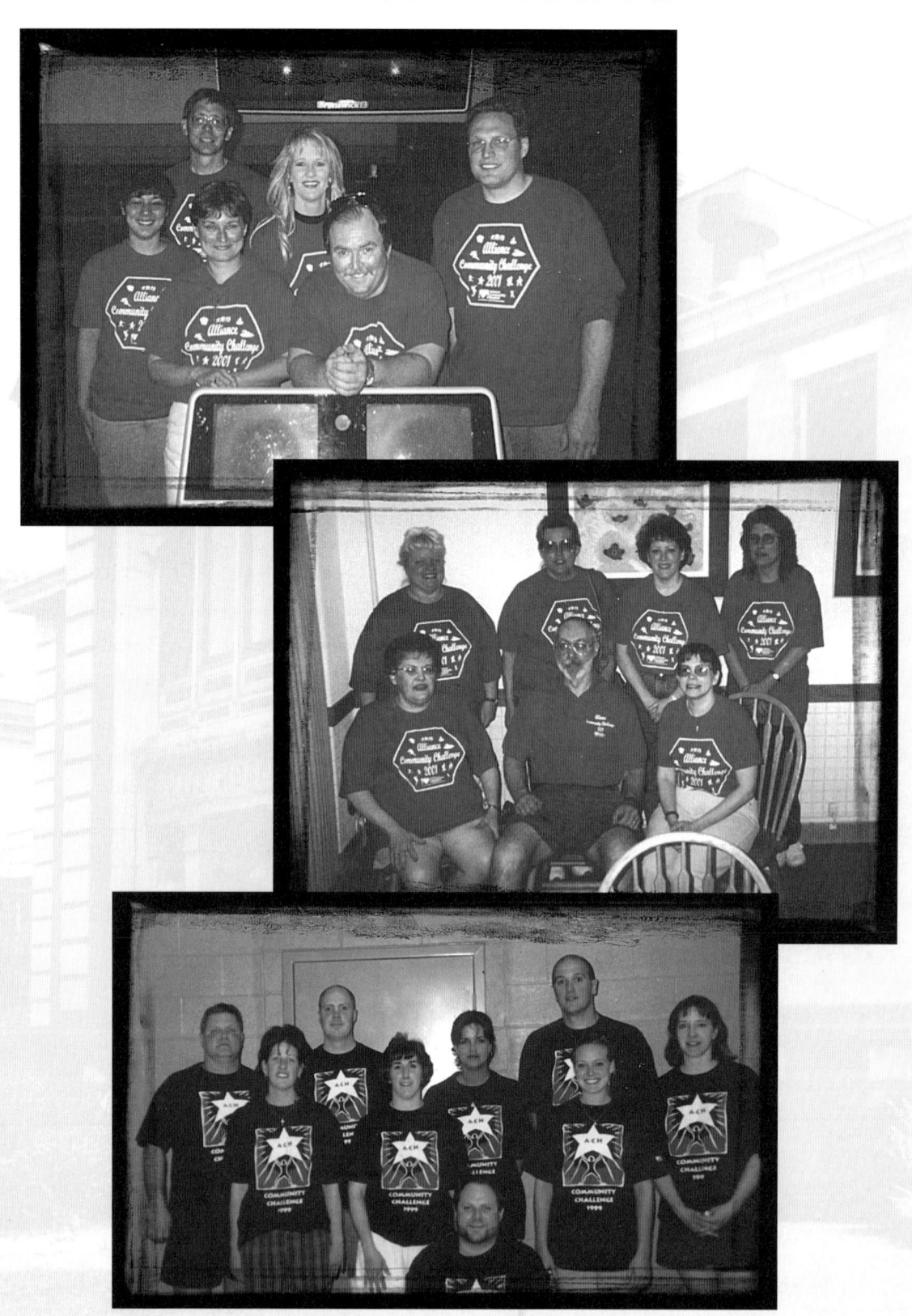

118 · *Photo Gallery* A CENTURY OF CARING

COLLEAGUES

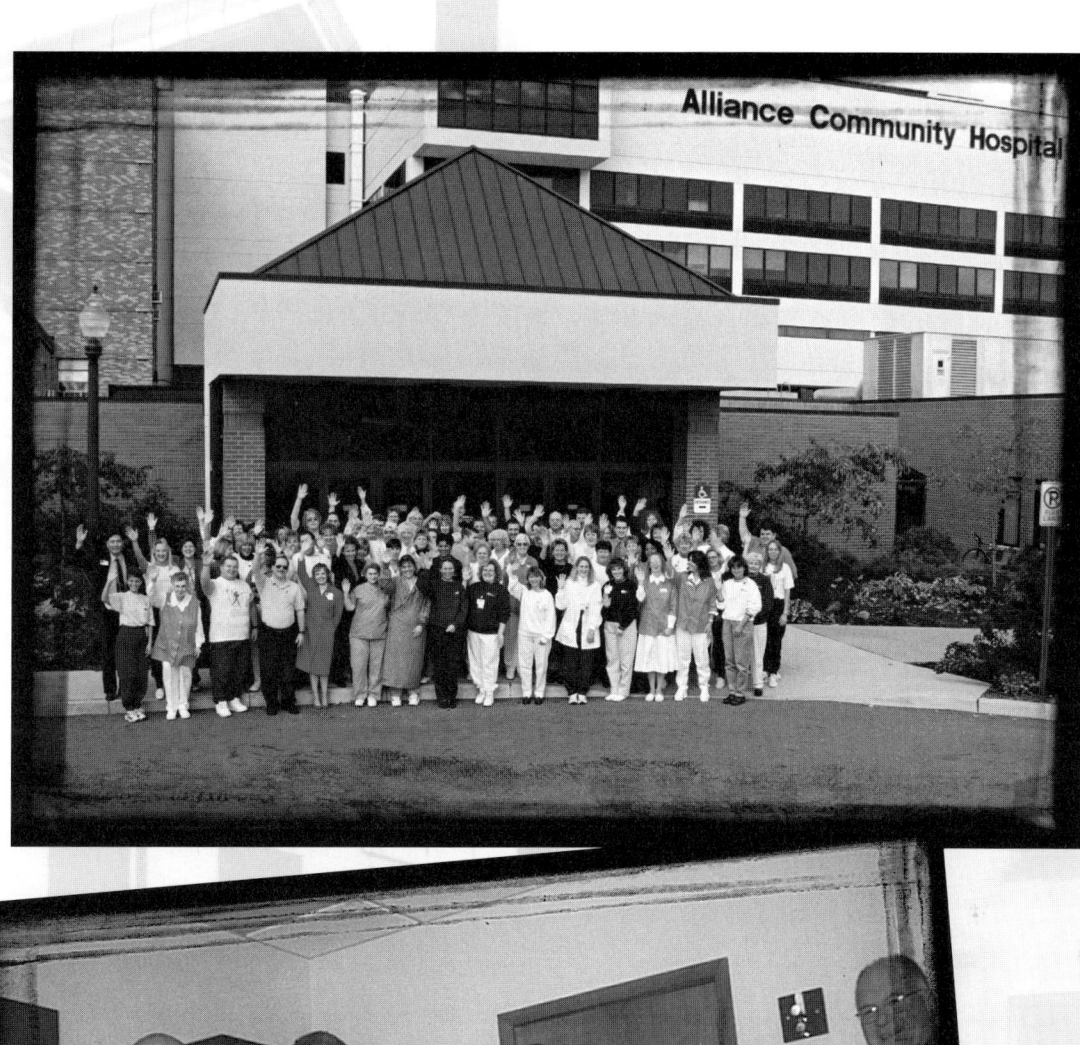

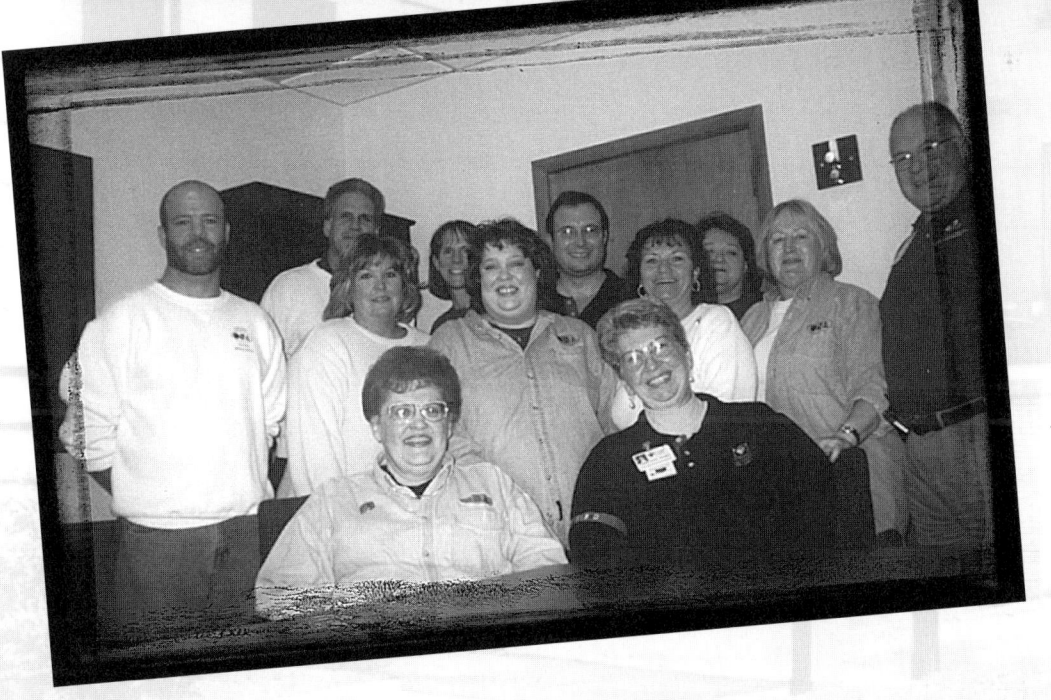

A CENTURY OF CARING *Photo Gallery* · 119

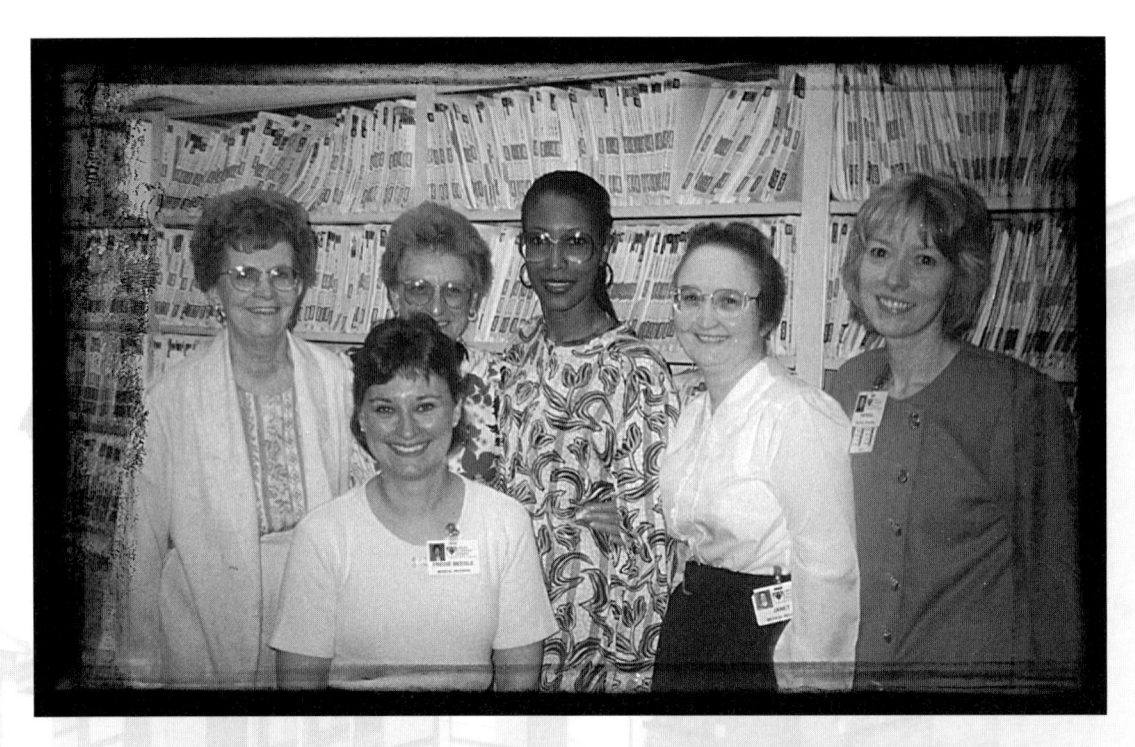

COLLEAGUES

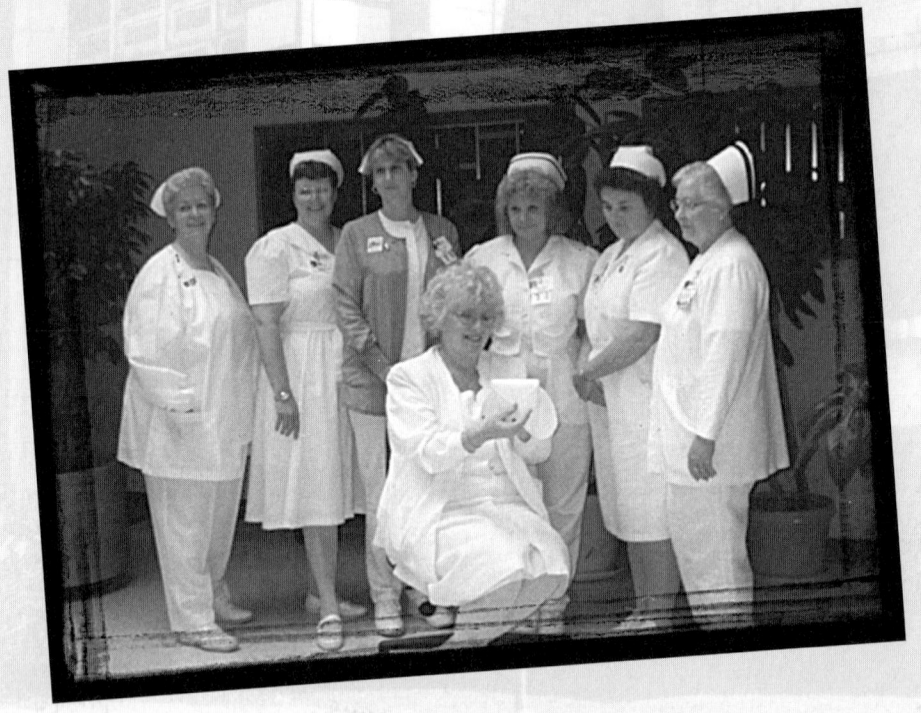

120 · *Photo Gallery*   A CENTURY OF CARING

COLLEAGUES

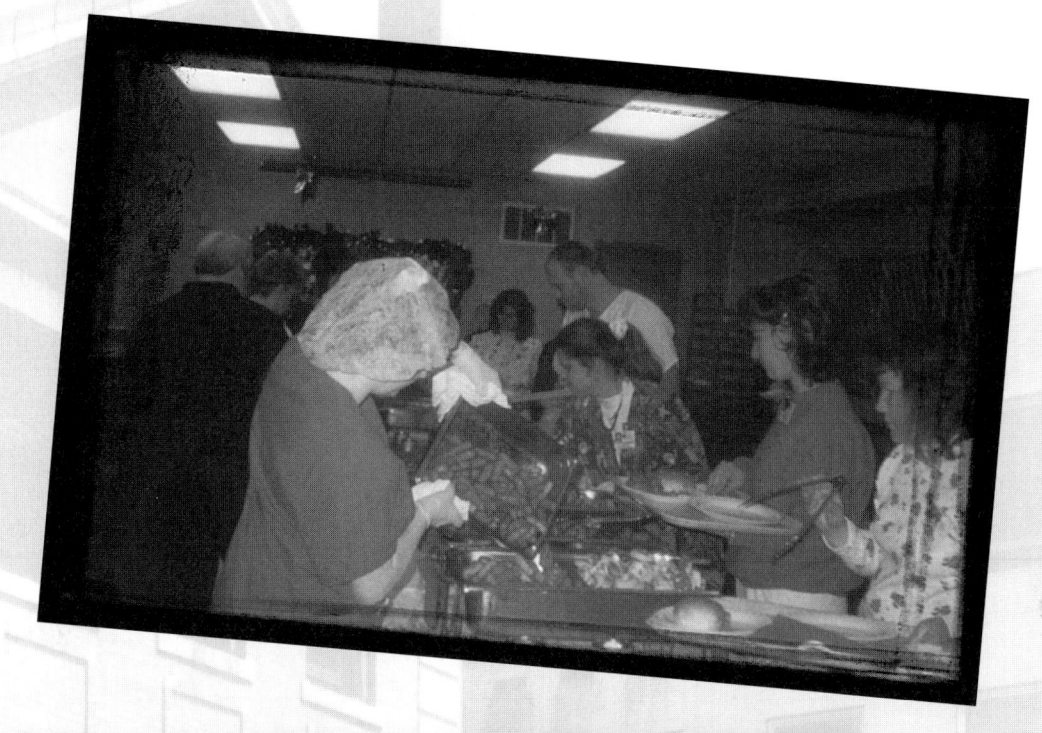

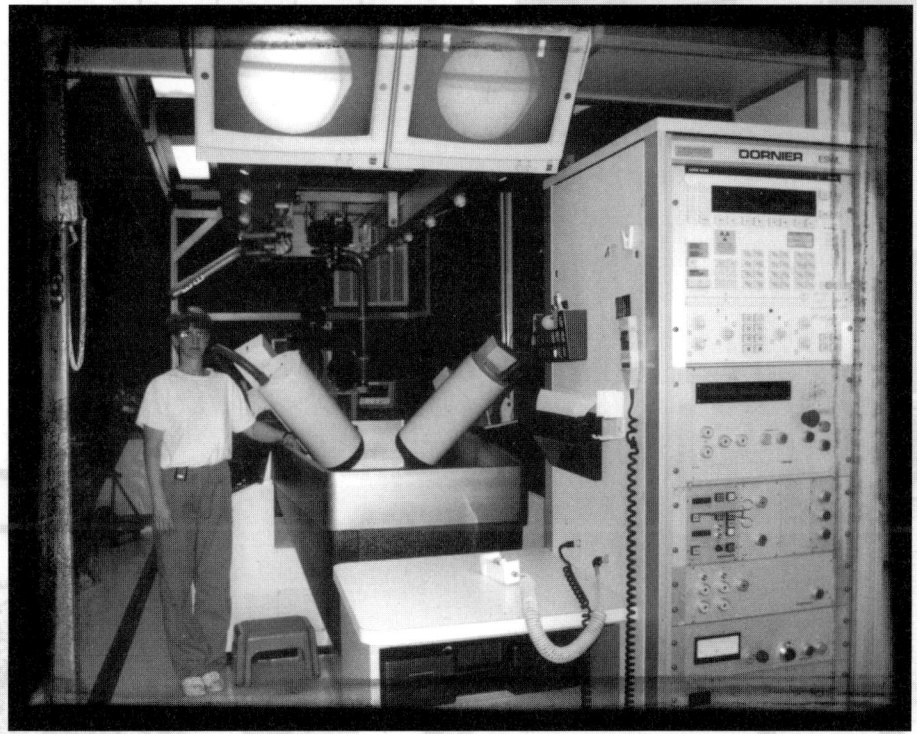

A CENTURY OF CARING *Photo Gallery* · 121

CELEBRATING 100 YEARS

122 · *Photo Gallery* A CENTURY OF CARING

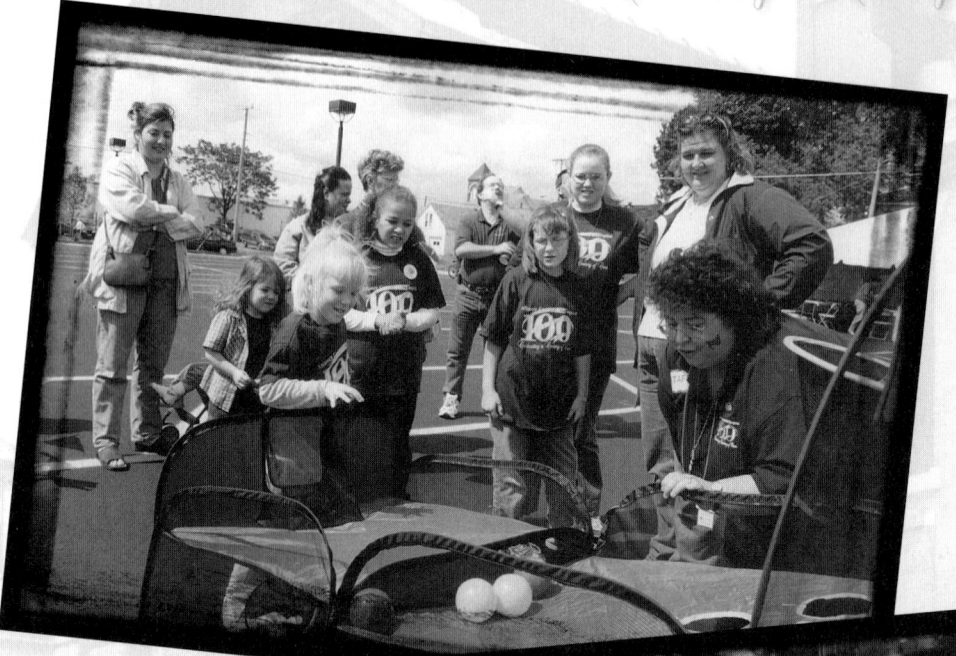

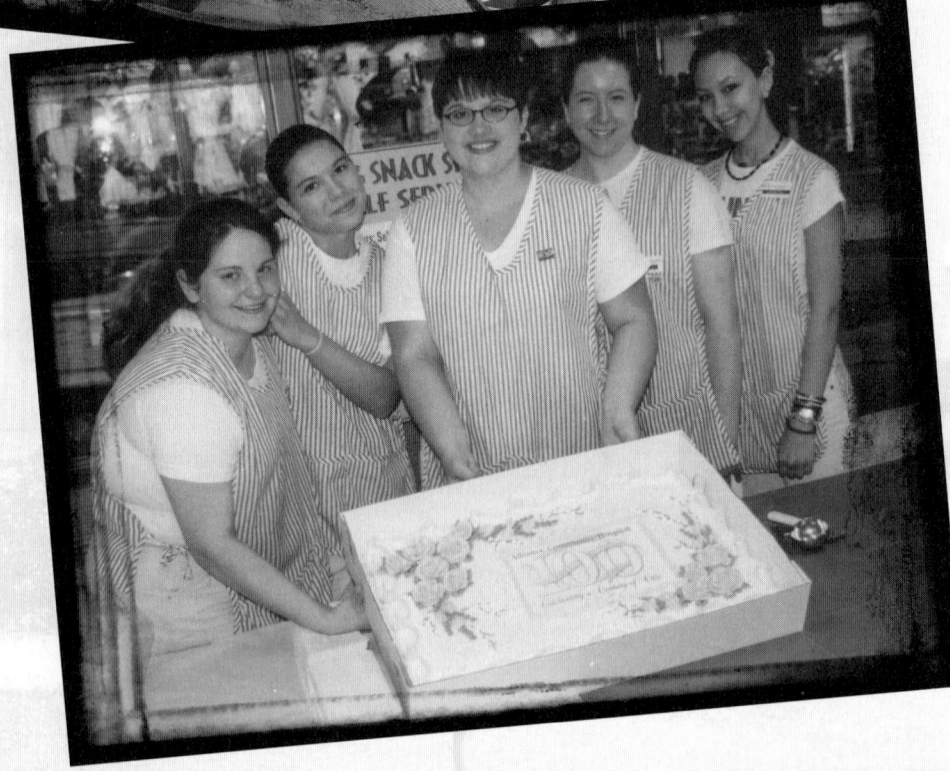

A CENTURY OF CARING *Photo Gallery* · 123

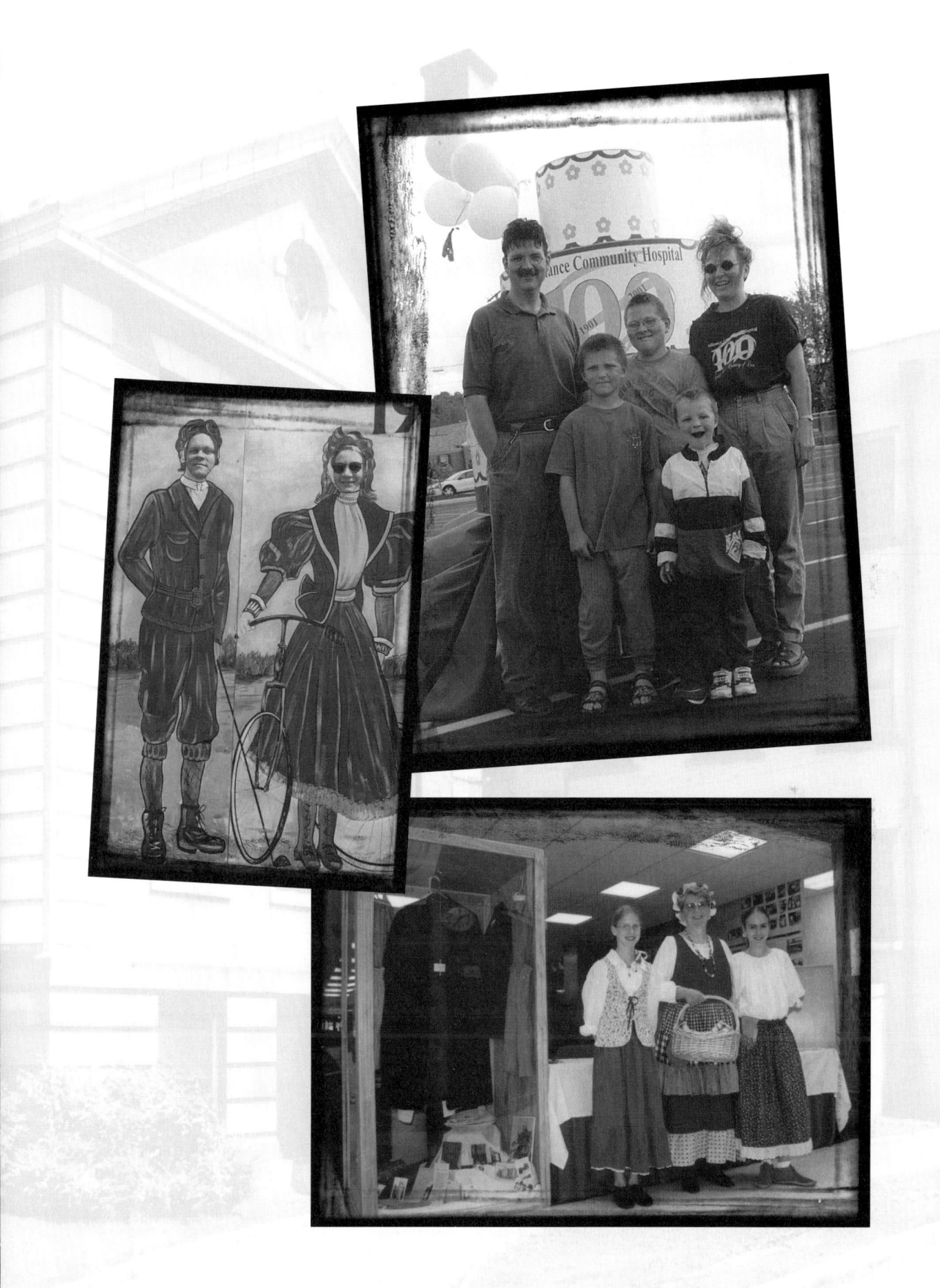

APPENDIX 1

The Deaconess Movement in America[210]

The Deaconess movement in modern history arose during the time of the Protestant Reformation and the French Revolution. We owe much of what we have come to know as the Deaconess movement to the interesting relationship between John Wesley, the founder of the Methodist church, and the German Lutheran church.

In the last decades of the eighteenth century a powerful religious movement arose in England. It united a variety of Christian faiths in their desire to help the needy. This is cited by Golder as the

> *first time [that] members ... of all denominations, including even the Quakers, united in common efforts for the promotion of the Kingdom of God. In a single decade some of the most important religious societies of our times were organized for this purpose, — in 1795, the London Missionary Society; in 1799, the Tract Society; in 1804, the British and foreign Bible Society.*

These religious societies connected with what Golder calls "women's societies ... for amelioration of suffering," which had sprung up during the Napoleonic wars, to form the modern Deaconess movement as we know it. Eventually these societies were joined together in a loose coalition that was originally patterned after the Roman Catholic Sisters of Mercy.

According to its founder, the German Lutheran Amelia Sieveking, the Protestant Sisters of Mercy was to be a "suitable calling for that class of single women who had no domestic duties and who spent their time in an unprofitable manner." After a terrible outbreak of cholera in Hamburg, Germany in 1831 Sieveking disbanded the Sisterhood (due mainly to the scorn she felt from the male doctors). Her lasting impact on our story can be seen in what Golder calls her ability to induce other women "to devote their gifts and energies to the service of suffering humanity." As we will see, this willingness to suffer humanity lies right at the core of the Deaconess philosophy.

The founder of the contemporary Deaconess movement was Pastor Theodore Fliedner who, during a tour of England and Holland in an attempt to raise money for his failing church in Kasierswerth, Germany, noticed that the English and the Dutch had "a number of benevolent institutions for the care of body and soul, — schools and educational institutions, asylums for the poor, the orphans, and the sick…." This so impressed him that upon his return to Germany, Fliedner founded the Kaiserswerth Deaconess House and opened it on October 13, 1836.[211] By the time of the 50th anniversary of the Kaiserswerth home, there were Deaconess Homes throughout Europe as well as in Jerusalem, Constantinople, Smyrna, Alexandria, Beirut, and Cairo.[212]

The first Deaconess Hospital and Home in America was founded in 1849 by Reverend Dr. W.A. Passavant. Its first patients were men returning from the Mexican War. The first Deaconesses were two women trained in Kaiserswerth by Fliedner himself. The first American Deaconess was Katharine Louise Martens, who was consecrated in May of 1850. She later went on to help found and eventually run the Deaconess Home and Hospital in Jacksonville, Illinois.[213]

APPENDIX 2
From the Diary of Mrs. M.E. Whitmore

Much of the best information about the early days of the hospital comes from the diary of the Reverend Kilmer's mother-in-law, Mrs. Whitmore. Evidently she lived in the Whitacre house while the Deaconess Home was being finished. (She served as, on and off, a nurse and/or supervisor of nurses). Her diary contains much mundane information about the hospital's earliest days (who was coming and going, what she ate, the health of her family, etc.). Below are some selections.

January 4, 1901: Miss Williams, daughter of Senator Williams, came to the home to select a room which she intended furnishing. The house contains three iron beds, a small parlor-cook, the Dauntless, a table, a desk with a broken leg, a bookcase of books, three stands, the smallest holding a bouquet of large white carnations, a few chairs, an old bureau, and some dishes and cooking utensils.

January 8, 1901: [F]ire started in the furnace, and the house was warm for the first time. … The water was turned on and we no longer have to go to our neighbors or even to the cellar, as formerly, for water.

January 9, 1901: The new kitchen range came today, also Mr. Kilmer bought washtub and bard, flour and other necessaries. Mr. Cassady donated three new beds.

January 10, 1901: The new telephone was put in today. The first message I received was that my mother was very ill. We cleaned some of the rooms today.

January 14, 1901: Our first patient was brought to the Hospital. His foot was crushed by the train running over it. His name is Patrick Gilhully. … We had a meeting of the ladies of Alliance in the interest of the Hospital at the Reformed Church [Immanuel] this afternoon. All are ready to help.

January 16, 1901: A new patient, Mr. Chas Stoll, of our church. Is very nervous. Has grip and Doctor fears Typhoid fever. Both patients are doing well.

January 22, 1901: Mrs. Granger sent granite ware, quite a lot, tinware and spiders. … This morning I asked God to send us a tea-pot. This evening when I returned, it was here, given by Mrs. Wilson. $12 came today for the Hospital and Home.

February 10, 1901: Mr. Stoll died at 4 o'clock this morning of typhoid fever. His sister was with him for a couple of days, and was a great comfort to him. He died very happy.

February 19, 1901: A Mr. W.H. Lee was brought into the Hospital supposed to be drugged by robbers on train, about 2 o'clock a.m. He came from California and was on his way home near Steubenville, O. He left this evening at 5 o'clock.

April 17, 1901: A public opening was held. There were quite a number of people here, and they realized a nice little sum.

APPENDIX 3
Alliance Citizens Health Association
PRESIDENTS 1986-PRESENT

1986 Charles Grove
1987 Charles Grove
1988 Charles Grove
1989 Charles Grove
1990 Randall Hunt
1991 Randall Hunt
1992 David Becker
1993 David Becker
1994 David Becker
1995 David Becker
1996 David Becker
1997 Scott Ingledue
1998 Scott Ingledue
1999 Scott Ingledue
2000 Scott Ingledue

APPENDIX 4
Alliance Community Hospital Foundation
PRESIDENTS 1986-PRESENT

1986 Randall Hunt
1987 Andrew Marhevsky
1988 Scott Ingledue
1989 Scott Ingledue
1990 Scott Ingledue
1991 Scott Ingledue
1992 Scott Ingledue
1993 Scott Ingledue
1994 Scott Ingledue
1995 Scott Ingledue
1996 Scott Ingledue
1997 David Bitonte, DO
1998 David Bitonte, DO
1999 Daniel Davia
2000 Daniel Davia

APPENDIX 5
AUXILIARY PRESIDENTS

Mrs. Harry Roderick · 1935-40
Miss Barbara Turkle · 1940-41
Mrs. Floyd Stamp · 1941-42
Mrs. H.L. Weaver · 1942-43
Mrs. Homer Scranton · 1943-44
Mrs. William M. Morgan · 1944-45
Mrs. George Donaldson · 1945-48
Mrs. M.T. Hunter · 1948-49

Mrs. J.L. McClintock · 1950-51

Mrs. P.K. Singer · 1950-51

Mrs. J.J. Hurst · 1951-53

Mrs. Guy Hoover · 1953-54

Mrs. Douglass King · 1954-58

Mrs. Merritt Crouch · 1958-60

Mrs. William Breckner · 1960-62

Mrs. Rollo Wileman · 1962-63

Mrs. Ralph Cole · 1963-65

Mrs. Nile Long · 1965-67

Mrs. Donald Barnhart · 1967

Mrs. George Bica · 1967

Mrs. H.D. Thomas · 1968-69

Mrs. Harold Harsh · 1969-71

Mrs. Wade Parkinson · 1971-73

Mrs. Kenneth Wable · 1973-75

Mrs. Milton Geiger · 1975-77

Mrs. Paul Stillwell · 1977-79

Mrs. Fred Burmeister · 1979-80

Mrs. Robert DeForest · 1980-81

Mrs. Scott Patterson · 1981-82

Mrs. Duane Wamsley · 1982-83

Mrs. John Benincasa · 1983-85

Mrs. Oscar Andreani · 1985-87

Mrs. William Bingham · 1987-88

Mrs. Claire Stahl · 1988-91

Mrs. Robert Connell · 1991-93

Mr. Alex Smith · 1993-95

Mrs. Ferne Phillips · 1995-97

Mrs. Evelyn Deuvall · 1997-01

[1] Blue, Herbert. *History of Stark County Ohio: Volume I.* Chicago: S.J. Clarke Publishing, 1928. 744.

[2] Looking through the *Alliance Review* for materials for this history, I noticed that water quality has been an ongoing concern nearly every year for the past 100 years.

[3] There is a good history of the first fifty years of the Auxiliary available from the hospital.

[4] Golder, Rev. C. *The History of The Deaconess Movement in the Christian Church.* Cincinnati: Jennings & Pye, 1903.

[5] *Alliance Daily Review.* Vol. 12 Issue 238.

[6] W.H. Ramsey, Vice-President; C.O. Waltz, Secretary; J.A. Boyd, Treasurer; C.W. Hemings, Auditor; Ms. Margaret Ubert, Head Nurse. See "The hospital Will be Known as the Deaconess Home." *Alliance Daily Review.* 18 January 1900.

[7] Much of the information about the founding of the hospital is sketchy. Most of the information in this first chapter comes from histories of the hospital contained within the hospital's own archive. There are no authors listed. Other helpful information comes from *History of Immanuel Reformed Church of Alliance, Ohio* by William Yerlan, and the *Alliance Review.*

[8] Blue, Herbert. *History of Stark County Ohio: Volume I.* Chicago: S.J. Clarke Publishing, 1928. 744.

[9] From the papers of Mrs. M.E. Whitmore, in the Alliance Community Hospital Archives.

[10] "It is Bought: The Whitacre Property for Use as a Hospital." *Alliance Daily Review.* 8 December 1900.

[11] From the papers of Mrs. M.E. Whitmore, in the Alliance Community Hospital Archives.

[12] *History of the Deaconess Movement in the Christian Church* 267-8.

[13] There is conflicting information about the number of beds in the early Deaconess Home. Most of the information from the *Review* and from early histories of Stark County indicate there were twenty beds of some sort.

[14] I am skeptical of this information if only because Golder's dates and statistics (i.e., the amount of money spent on the initial property, etc.) do not agree with *any* available local information.

[15] Golder 472.

[16] *Alliance Daily Review Special Edition: Industrial.* 28 July 1906.

[17] Ibid.

[18] "Alliance City Hospital Stockholders Meeting." *Alliance Daily Review.* 11 January 1908.

[19] "The Hospital: When it was organized, and by whom." *Alliance Daily Review.* 29 May 1906.

[20] Indeed, one of the difficulties that I encountered when researching the years 1910-1920 was that the building of a new hospital, while important locally, was hardly on par with the declaration of war by England or the sinking of the Lusitania by Germany, thus what would have been front-page news any other time was buried because of all of the national and international events of the age.

[21] *Alliance Review.* June 4, 1914.

[22] As far as I can tell this is not the same organization that is now the Hospital Auxiliary.

[23] "City Hospital To Be Turned Over Thursday." *Alliance Daily Review and Leader.* 12 September 1916.

[24] "Need of Help for Hospital." *Alliance Daily Review and Leader.* 19 September 1916.

[25] Hospital Filled; Patient Suffers." *Alliance Daily Review and Leader.* 29 September 1916.

[26] "Hospital will be finished at once." *Alliance Daily Review and Leader.* 3 October 1916.

[27] "Need Nurses at Hospital." *Alliance Daily Review and Leader.* 20 January 1917.

[28] "City Hospital now Complete." *Alliance Daily Review and Leader.* 21 February 1917.

[29] "Twins Born Two Days Apart; Unique Operations are Used." *Alliance Review and Leader.* 1 November 1917.

[30] "Christmas Tree at City Hospital Brings Cheer." *Alliance Daily Review and Leader.* 27 December 1919.

[31] Will Complete Hospital with Funds Available." *Alliance Review.* 11 January 1922.

[32] *Alliance Review.* 1 February 1922.

[33] "National Hospital Day Will Be Celebrated in Alliance on May 12th." *Alliance Review.* 3 May 1922.

[34] "Boost in Rates At Hospital is Proposed Here." *Alliance Review.* 8 July 1922.

[35] "Eighty-Five Surgical Cases Treated at City Hospital Last Month." *Alliance Review.* 30 September 1922.

[36] "Propose Changes in Management of City Hospital." *Alliance Review.* 17 October 1922.

[37] "Hospital is Warm Center of Debate at Solons' Meet." *Alliance Review.* 3 October 1922.

[38] "Legislation for $42,000 bond issue is enacted." *Alliance Review.* 24 October 1922.

[39] "Praise work of Hospital Head Who is Leaving City." *Alliance Review.* 30 December 1922.

[40] "Will Start Campaign of Financing $2,500,00 NovoPathic Hospital, To Be Built in Alliance, Monday." *Alliance Review.* 26 May 1922.

[41] It's important to remember, however, that it is now June and the hospital had promised that it would be done with the addition in April.

[42] "Will Equip New Annex At Hospital Right Away." *Alliance Review.* 13 June 1922.

[43] "Open Proposals for Hospital Supplies Here." *Alliance Review.* 2 October 1923.

[44] "New Hospital Equipment is Purchased Here." *Alliance Review.* 13 November 1923.

[45] "Alliance City Hospital Cuts Into Yearly Deficit in 1923." *Alliance Review.* 2 February 1924.

[46] "Give Rotary Club Hospital Wing for Children's Ward." *Alliance Review.* 6 February 1924.

[47] "Auditor Halts Bond Issue to Fix Hospital." *Alliance Review.* 3 March 1925.

[48] "City Must Foot Repair bill at Hospital." *Alliance Review.* 13 March 1925.

[49] "To Split cost of Hospital Repairs." *Alliance Review.* 17 March 1925.

[50] "Cultures at Cost, is Hospital Plan." *Alliance Review.* 19 March 1925.

[51] "Dr. Albert Wild Central Figure in Court Fight." *Alliance Review.* 18 April 1925.

[52] "City Hospital Heads Called For Contempt." *Alliance Review.* 22 April 1925.

[53] "'Closed Ring' is Charge of Dr. Wild in Court Fight." *Alliance Review.* 28 April 1925.

[54] "Hospital Clash Still in Court." *Alliance Review.* 29 April 1925. For complete copies of both the plaintiff's and the defendant's closing briefs, see "Decision This Week in Hospital Fight," *Alliance Review.* 5 May 1925.

[55] "City Hospital Case in Hands of Judge." *Alliance Review.* 9 May 1925.

[56] "Suspension of Wild to Stand, Court Rules." *Alliance Review.* 12 May 1925. The entire text of the court's decision, nearly 20 pages, is reprinted in this article.

[57] "Doctor to Carry Hospital Fight to Higher Court." *Alliance Review.* 13 May 1925.

[58] "Offer Wild Hospital Rights." *Alliance Review.* 19 May 1925.

[59] "Spurs Peace Offer in Hospital Fight." *Alliance Review.* 21 May 1925.

[60] Unfortunately, the stock market crash in October 1929 soon put an end to Alliance's dreams of airplane manufacturing.

[61] All of these were recommended by the Ohio Department of Health.

[62] "Stress Need for Hospital Annex." *Alliance Review.* 12 January 1927.

[63] "City Hospital Closes Year with Deficit." *Alliance Review.* 19 January 1927.

[64] "Face Deficit in Operating Revenue Here." *Alliance Review.* 25 January 1927.

[65] "Service to Mankind is Key note at Graduation." *Alliance Review.* 28 May 1927.

[66] "Complete Work on New Improvements at City Hospital." *Alliance Review.* 27 June 1927.

[67] "City Pruned Hospital Fund Down too Fine." *Alliance Review.* 2 August 1927. Interestingly enough, another item that was cut from the budget at the same city council meeting was Silver Park's bandstand. This would cause a scandal, including the resignation of the entire parks board.

[68] "First Six Months Best in Hospital History." *Alliance Review.* 2 August 1927.

[69] "Forty Nurses Now on Hospital Staff." *Alliance Review.* 1 September 1927.

[70] "Alliance City Hospital On Approved List." *Alliance Review.* 7 October 1927.

[71] "Death Rate Drops at City Hospital." *Alliance Review.* 18 January 1928.

[72] "Hospital School Warmly Praised by State Expert." *Alliance Review.* 26 October 1928.

[73] "Claim Radio is Hospital Need." *Alliance Review.* 21 April 1928.

[74] "Purchase X-ray Equipment for City Hospital." *Alliance Review.* 9 October 1928.

[75] "City Hospital Report Reflects Busy Year." *Alliance Review.* 25 January 1929.

[76] "Alliance Hospital is Pronounced Safe." *Alliance Review.* 16 May 1929.

[77] "Alliance City Hospital on Approved List." *Alliance Review.* 19 November 1929. An interesting part of the story: it was reported that at the annual staff meeting, a session was held on "medico-legal" issues … perhaps an indication of what the future would hold for hospitals throughout the country?

[78] In doing the research for this book I was flabbergasted at some of the attempts by the Federal government to get out of the early depression—floating bonds, having people in cities that had money donate to cities that didn't, and increasing taxes despite the fact that people couldn't pay what they already owed.

[79] An interesting example of this is the ill-fated history of the Alliance Aircraft Factory which had been planned, proposed, and opened to wide acclaim in 1928-9. After receiving orders for its first five planes, the company decided to float an initial public offering of stock in the amount of $250,000 on October 1, 1929. Twenty-eight days later the company was in ruins, its valuation at roughly 10% of what it had been at the beginning of the month.

[80] "Alliance is Chosen for Nurses' Meeting." *Alliance Review.* 29 January 1930.

[81] "To Rush Man Into Office." *Alliance Review.* 28 February 1930.

[82] "Hospital Day Marks Opening of Book Drive." *Alliance Review.* 10 May 1930.

[83] "Hospital Library Drive is Closed." *Alliance Review.* 17 May 1930.

[84] "Use Footprints to Tag Hospital Babies." *Alliance Review.* 20 August 1930. The Bamberger-Watkins case was a nationally covered "switched baby" case.

[85] *Alliance Review.* 25 August 1930.

[86] "New York Man to Head Hospital." *Alliance Review.* 16 September 1930.

[87] "'Give a dollar' is Appeal in Hospital Fund Drive." *Alliance Review.* 30 September 1930.

[88] *Alliance Review.* 17 October 1930.

[89] "Need Better Home Facilities for Hospital Nurses." *Alliance Review.* 2 December 1930.

[90] *Alliance Review.* 5 December 1930.

[91] "Need $9,750 to Operate Hospital." *Alliance Review.* 13 December 1930.

[92] "Council Heeds Hospital Appeal." *Alliance Review.* 20 December 1930.

[93] "Change Looms at City Hospital." *Alliance Review.* 5 January 1931.

[94] "City Closes 1930 Books Short $5,886." *Alliance Review.* 8 January 1931.

[95] "Pick Hospital Superintendent." *Alliance Review.* 13 January 1931.

[96] "Tells Council Why Hospital Loses Money." *Alliance Review.* 17 February 1931.

[97] *Alliance Review.* 1 April 1931.

[98] "'Hospital Day' Draws Throng of Visitors." *Alliance Review.* 13 May 1931.

[99] *Alliance Review.* 25 & 28 May 1931.

[100] "Solicitor Ordered to Collect Bills." *Alliance Review.* 16 June 1931.

[101] "To Reject Patients Until Bills are Paid." *Alliance Review.* 7 July 1931.

[102] "Hospital to Lose $1,500 on Mishaps." *Alliance Review.* 6 August 1931.

[103] For more on the levy, see *Alliance Review.* 18 August 1931. For information on the nursing school see *Alliance Review.* 17 September 1931.

[104] "City Hospital Lives Within 1931 Income." *Alliance Review.* 8 December 1931.

[105] "Four Members of Hospital Staff Resign." *Alliance Review.* 16 February 1932.

[106] "Nurses will Retain Posts at Hospital." *Alliance Review.* 17 February 1932.

[107] "General Pay Slash Seems Inevitable for City Employees." *Alliance Review.* 14 February 1932.

[108] *Alliance Review.* 19 April 1932.

[109] "Practice Economy at City Hospital." *Alliance Review.* 17 May 1932.

[110] "3 Members of Nursing Staff Resign." *Alliance Review.* 12 August 1932.

[111] "Quits Women's Club to take Hospital Job." *Alliance Review.* 18 August 1932.

[112] "Urge Closing of Training School Here." *Alliance Review.* 20 December 1932. Other cost-cutting measures considered at the same city council meeting included shutting down the #2 (South Liberty) firehouse, the elimination of the council clerk's salary, and the move to hold elections in "rent free" buildings.

[113] "Head: 'Want Hospital out of City Politics.'" *Alliance Review.* 30 December 1932.

[114] Wagner had resigned on 31 December of the previous year in keeping with the city's new budget plan in which all city employees would have to resign and be reappointed by the mayor and/or council.

[115] "Hospital is center of Long Discussion at Solons' Session." *Alliance Review.* 4 January 1933.

[116] "Hospital Plan Hits Snag." *Alliance Review.* 6 January 1933.

[117] "Council Votes Down Measure to Suspend Training of Nurses." *Alliance Review.* 12 January 1933.

[118] "Council Creates New City Hospital Position." *Alliance Review.* 6 February 1934.

[119] "Montague Names Hospital Finance Director." *Alliance Review.* 16 March 1934.

[120] To be fair, however, it is important to remember that nearly everything in Alliance, including the city government, the schools, Mount Union college, and most of the businesses were insolvent.

[121] "Study Situation at Hospital." *Alliance Review.* 30 January 1935.

[122] "Hospital Finance Director is Appointed." *Alliance Review.* 6 February 1935.

[123] "Rodeo will Raise Funds for Hospital." *Alliance Review.* 11 September 1935.

[124] "Hospital in Need of Fresh Supplies." *Alliance Review.* 14 September 1935.

[125] "Plenty of Thrills for Rodeo Audience." *Alliance Review.* 18 September 1935.

[126] *Alliance Review.* 15 October 1935.

[127] "Stress Place of Hospital in Community." *Alliance Review.* 1 November 1935.

[128] "Mathematicians are still 'Struggling' over Hospital vote." *Alliance Review.* 7 November 1935.

[129] "$55,672 is Collected at Hospital." *Alliance Review.* 11 January 1936.

[130] *Alliance Hospital Auxiliary: The First Fifty Years.* Publication of the Alliance Community Hospital Auxiliary.

[131] "Hospital Levy Added to June Tax Billing." *Alliance Review.* 14 May 1936.

[132] "Hospital Levy ruled off Tax Duplicates." *Alliance Review.* 30 June 1936.

[133] "Will Not Contest Hospital Ruling." *Alliance Review.* 1 July 1936.

[134] "Ask Share of Carey Fund to Aid Hospital." *Alliance Review.* 6 August 1936.

[135] "Seek New Funds to Avoid Hospital Deficit." *Alliance Review.* 8 December 1936.

[136] $2,828,905 Asked for WPA Projects." *Alliance Review.* 6 September 1936; "11 Concerns Seek Nurses' Home Work." *Alliance Review.* 4 March 1937.

[137] "State Board Asks Changes at Hospital." *Alliance Review.* 16 November 1937.

[138] "City Hospital School Crisis is Averted." *Alliance Review.* 14 December 1937.

[139] "Will Slash City Payroll to Avert Crisis." *Alliance Review.* 15 March 1938.

[140] "Bond Issue is Approved by Council." *Alliance Review.* 8 June 1939.

[141] "City Hospital School Given High Rating." *Alliance Review.* 18 April 1938.

[142] "Graduates of City Hospital Pass Ohio Exam." *Alliance Review.* 8 March 1938. "Hospital Class Will Get Pins Friday Night." *Alliance Review.* 22 June 1938. "City Hospital Will Graduate Class of Six." *Alliance Review.* 21 June 1939.

[143] At this point in the history I start using the Alliance Community Hospital's own archives for documentation. Many of the articles in said archives are undated. Some of the dates on the articles are handwritten and are not necessarily accurate. I have tried, whenever possible, to make clear when and where things happened.

[144] Much of this information comes from William Manchester's excellent book *the Glory and the Dream: A Narrative History of America: 1932-1974.* New York: Bantam Books, 1975.

[145] "Carr is War Appointee at Hospital." *Alliance Review.* 15 September 1942.

[146] *Alliance Review.* Date unknown.

[147] "City Hospital Regains Approved List Rating." *Alliance Review.* January 1943.

[148] "City Need for Larger Nurses Quarters Here." *Alliance Review.* 18 May 1943.

[149] "Financial Outlook for Hospital Called 'Definitely' Bad" and "Dr. G.L. King Cites Need for 60 Additional Hospital Beds." Both *Alliance Review.* Dates unknown.

[150] "Will Become Head of Nursing Staff." *Alliance Review.* Date unknown.

[151] "Reveal Long-Studied Plan to Place Hospital Under Direction of Trusteeship." *Alliance Review.* 10 February 1945. The "Alliance Betterment Council" was made up of representatives of every civic and fraternal organization in the city.

[152] "Lions Club Endorses City Hospital Plan." *Alliance Review.* Date unknown.

[153] "Oppose Plan." *Alliance Review.* 6 March 1945.

[154] "Open Forum." *Alliance Review.* 5 March 1945.

[155] "Hospital Plan Given Approval by Legion Post" 6 March; "Rotary Endorses Hospital Set Up" 8 March; "Mrs. Logan Tent Approves City Hospital Transfer" 4 March; "Hospital Change Approved by Sons of Veterans" 3 March; "Legion Women Endorse City Hospital Plan"; "Vets' Auxiliary Approves Hospital Trusteeship Plan"; "Doctors Wives"; All in *Alliance Review.* Dates unknown.

[156] "Well Matured Plan." *Alliance Review.* 12 April 1945.

[157] "Open Forum." *Alliance Review.* 6 March; 21 March; 10 April; 18 April.

[158] "Dean of Pennsylvania Graduate School of Medicine Made City Hospital Survey." *Alliance Review.* 2 April 1945; "Non-Profit Organization For

Hospital In Line With Expert's Recommendations." *Alliance Review.* 7 April 1945; "Hospital at 'Crossroads' Dr. Buerki Says in Report." *Alliance Review.* 5 April 1945; "Suggests 140-Bed Hospital to Meet Alliance's Needs." *Alliance Review.* 9 April 1945.

[159] "Opens Way for Trusteeship." *Alliance Review.* 18 June 1945.

[160] "Open Letter to the People of Alliance." *Alliance Review.* Date unknown.

[161] "Notice!" Paid Political Advertisement. *Alliance Review.* 18 July 1945.

[162] "Levy and Hospital Trusteeship Approved." *Alliance Review.* Date Unknown. One interesting note about this election: the one mayoral candidate who was in favor of the move to trusteeship, Democrat Robert Althouse, was voted into office in the same election.

[163] "'Put it Over' Becomes Challenge in Canvass to Expand City Hospital." *Alliance Review.* Date unknown.

[164] "Hospital Must Expand to East, Workers Told." *Alliance Review.* Date unknown.

[165] "Dollars or Lives." *Alliance Review.* Date unknown.

[166] "Hospital Fund Nears Goal with Only $86,392 to go." *Alliance Review.* Date unknown.

[167] *Alliance Review.* Date and headline unknown.

[168] "New Hospital Assured." Paid advertisement. *Alliance Review.* Date unknown.

[169] "Raise $315,120 To Expand Hospital." *Alliance Review.* 11 February 1948.

[170] "Nurses Training to Stay At Hospital"; "Nurses To Be Capped At City Hospital"; "Will Retain Staff At City Hospital"; "Change At Hospital May Take 4 Months." *Alliance Review.* Dates unknown.

[171] "Dr. Perry F. King, Dean of City's Surgeons, Succumbs." *Alliance Review.* Date unknown.

[172] "Alliance Faces a Crisis." Pamphlet published by Alliance City Hospital. On file in the hospital's archives.

[173] "Get 'Go Ahead' on Hospital; Will Open Bids Next Month." *Alliance Review.* 4 October 1950.

[174] "Will Break Ground Soon for Hospital." *Alliance Review.* Date unknown.

[175] "Need $112,071 to Give City Complete Modern Hospital." *Alliance Review.* Date unknown.

[176] "Old Memories and Bricks Tumble Together in Nurses Home Razing." *Alliance Review.* 10 December 1949.

[177] "The Hospital Story." Unpublished MS, Alliance Community Hospital Archives.

[178] *Alliance Hospital Auxiliary: The First Fifty Years.* Publication of the Alliance Community Hospital Auxiliary.

[179] Notes from Carol Reed to Karen Vrabec and Larry Halm.

[180] "Hospital Opening Set July 31." *Alliance Review.* 23 July 1976.

[181] "Hospital to Buy Former Store." *Alliance Review.* Date Unknown.

[182] "Hospital board Approves Rate Increase, Fathers' Presence in Delivery Room." *Alliance Review.* Date unknown.

[183] "Letter to the Editor." *Alliance Review.* Date unknown.

[184] "Nurses Strike at Hospital." *Alliance Review.* 30 September 1976.

[185] "Maximum Care Expansion Reflects Community Need." *Alliance Review.* 27 January 1981.

[186] "Hospital Board Looks at Long Range Goals." *Alliance Review.* 29 April 1981.

[187] "Flower Shop Added at City Hospital." *Alliance Review*. 17 November 1982.

[188] "Hospital Planning Progresses." *Alliance Review*. 9 November 1982. I believe that Peters is referring to the 1917 building.

[189] "Medley Appointed acting chief officer at hospital." *Alliance Review*. 29 September 1982.

[190] "Wert takes post in Dayton." *Alliance Review*. 26 September 1982.

[191] "Hospital financial package receives tentative approval." *Alliance Review*. 21 September 1982.

[192] *Annual Report*. 1984.

[193] This information comes from unpublished notes from the 1985 Board meeting.

[194] All information about the new surgery comes from the 1985 *Annual Report*.

[195] All of this information comes from unpublished notes contained in the hospital's archives.

[196] 1987 *Annual Report*.

[197] 1994 *Annual Report*.

[198] 1995 *Annual Report*.

[199] Notes from Carol Reed to Karen Vrabec and Larry Halm.

[200] 1997 *Annual Report*.

[201] 1999 *Annual Report*.

[202] 1999 *Annual Report*.

[203] 1999 *Annual Report*.

[204] 2000 *Annual Report*.

[205] Personal interview with Stan Jonas. July 2001.

[206] "Alliance Hospital traces 100-year history." *Alliance Review*. 25 September 2001.

[207] "Frightened Residents Flood ER." *Alliance Review*. 29 May 2001.

[208] "Caution and Concern: Thousands of area residents get antibiotics; CDC may order vaccinations." *Alliance Review*. 4 June 2001

[209] "Beautiful People." *Alliance Review*. 4 June 2001.

[210] Most of the information in this essay comes from Golder, Rev. C. *The Deaconess Movement in the Christian Church.* Cincinnati: Jennings and Pye, 1903.

[211] Fliedner's story is a fascinating one – he also did pioneering work in the realm of prison reform and started the Rhenish-Westphalian Prison Society to improve not only prison conditions but conditions for prisoners upon release.

[212] Golder 68-74.

[213] Golder 252-4.

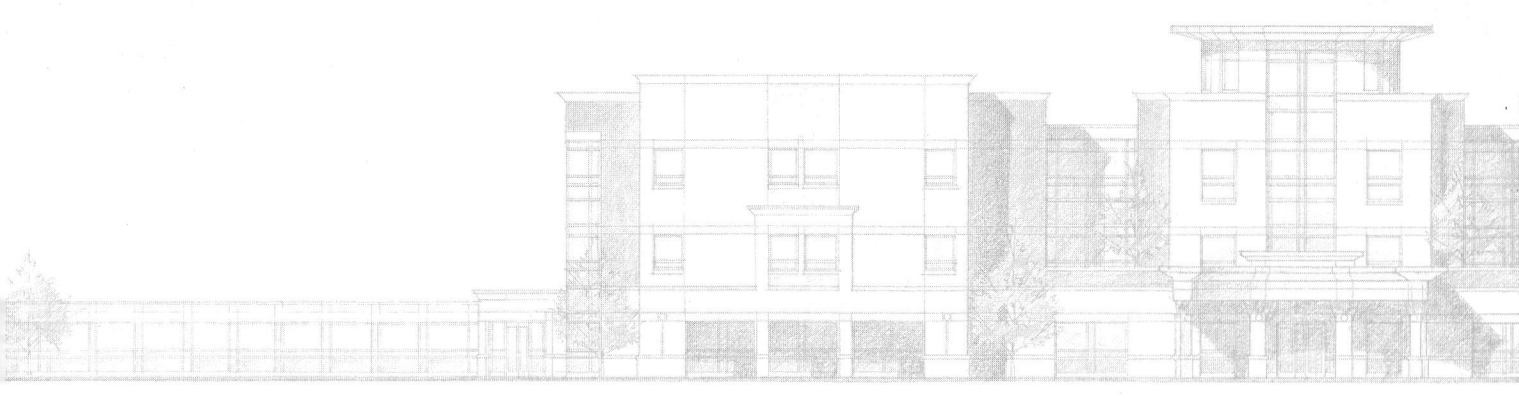

NORTH ELEVATION

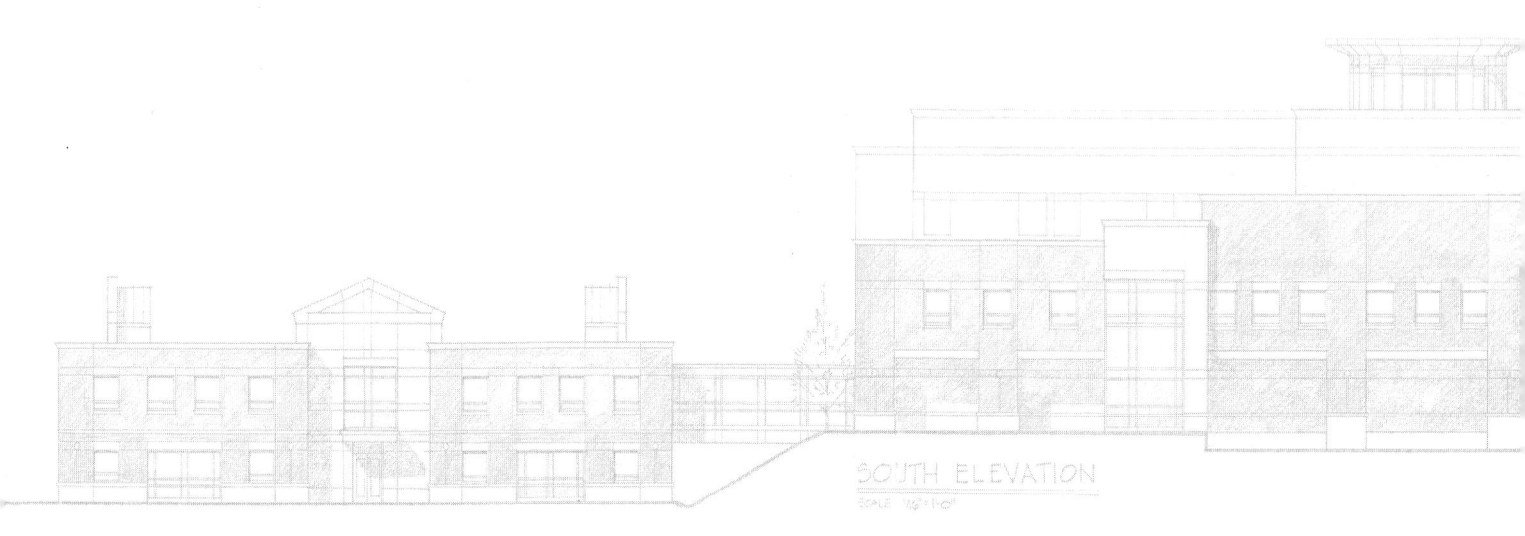

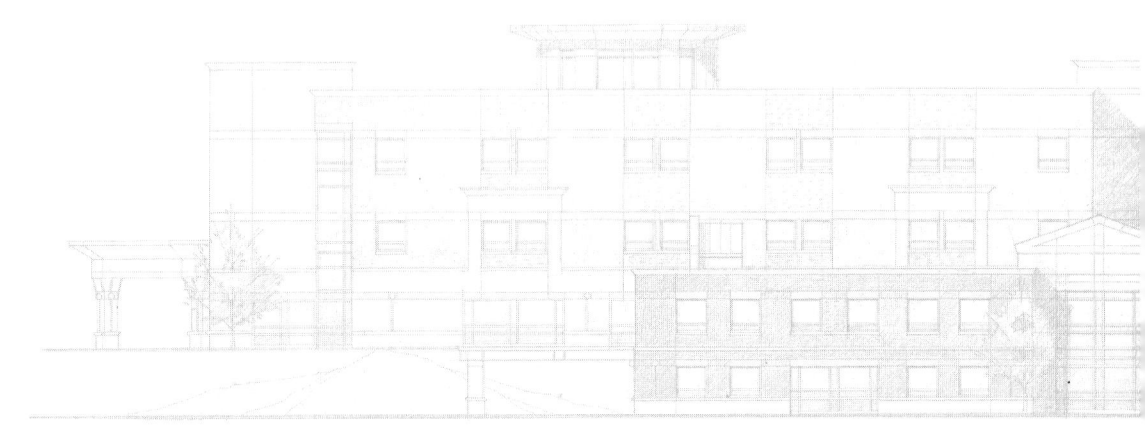

SOUTH ELEVATION

WEST ELEVATION

WEST ELEVATION - REAR

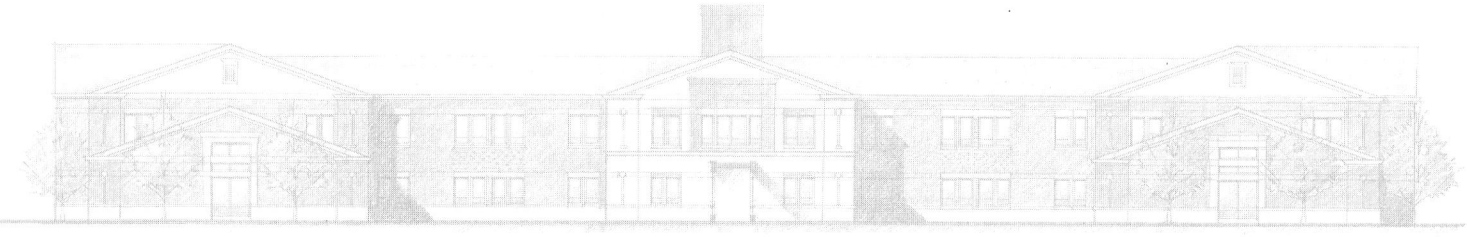